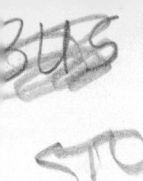

11-7-75

food reform:
our desperate need

FOOD REFORM: OUR DESPERATE NEED

BY ROBIN HUR

Heidelberg Publishers o Austin, Texas
1975

Published by Heidelberg Publishers, Inc.
3707 Kerbey Lane
Austin, Texas 78731

Library of Congress Cataloging in Publication Data

Hur, Robin.
  Food reform.
  Bibliography: p.
  1. Nutritionally induced diseases. I. Title.
RC622.H9   613.2   75–19083
ISBN 0–913206–05–9

1881229

contents

preface

By their late teens almost all North Americans and Europeans are plagued with fatty build-ups in their blood vessels (atherosclerosis) which serves as the root cause of heart attacks, strokes and other cardiovascular seizures. Atherosclerosis is responsible for the death of more North Americans than all other causes combined. Meat, eggs and dairy products are heavily laden with substances which promote this pathological condition.

Cancer of the bowel, breast cancer (and other female cancers), cancer of the pancreas, stomach cancer and cancer of the kidney and liver have all been linked to animal products and processed foods in the diet. The only major forms of cancer that have not been linked to specific food items in normal Western diets are associated with smoking, and the desire to smoke itself has been linked to meat-eating, dietary sugar and coffee.

Hypertension (high blood pressure) is ranked as the second biggest killer in the United States, and it is "normal" in the United States and Europe to experience rising blood pressure with age. High blood pressure can normally be cured in a short time by a salt-free, whole-foods vegetarian diet, yet the disease is now being treated with powerful drugs which are of questionable value as protection against hypertension-related disorders and which force patients to become permanently drug-dependent.

Diabetes and multiple sclerosis are widespread and growing rapidly in the wealthier nations where intake of sugar and fat is high. Both diseases are classified as incurable yet both diseases have been overcome by sugar-free, low-fat diets. The vast majority of the population in North America and Europe is above optimum weight, and obesity is a major factor in high blood pressure and diabetes. Obesity can be eradicated by high-carbohydrate diets.

Stooping backs, cataracts, impaired hearing, fragile bones and general debilitation are taken as inevitable aspects of "aging" in the West. Digestive problems afflict most aging Westerners and constipation, abdominal pain and hemorrhoids trouble vast numbers at every age. Every one of these conditions have been directly linked to meat-based diets. These afflictions are rare among groups taking sound near-vegetarian diets.

Deficiencies in our diets lead to nerve degeneration, brain damage and emotional disorders including anxiety, depression, irritability, insomnia, somnolence, fear, nervousness and a general lack of interest in life. Sugar, alcohol, coffee and hundreds of drugs also contribute to emotional disorders.

While deficiencies in the normal diets abound, the primary problem is excesses which include calories, fats (especially animal fats), salt, refined carbohydrates, medicines, caffeine, cholesterol, purines, bile acids, phosphorus and protein, *yes protein*! Advocates of supplements turn a blind eye to the fact that even if all the deficiencies in normal diets could be eliminated (which current supplements are ill-suited to achieve) there would be little, if any, let-up in our decline and degeneration. A carefully chosen mix of vitamins and minerals would no doubt benefit individuals who wish to continue to bombard their bodies with meat, eggs, sugar, refined foods, salt, drugs, coffee, oil, spices, cooking, smoking, etc., but it is imperative they be told the truth. The truth is that if they are to escape degenerative disease, they must change their way of eating. "Pill-pushers" are impeding necessary changes by promoting the destructive essence of meat-based diets: protein.

Advocates of high protein intake are speaking against a hundred years of research findings when they claim high protein boosts endurance, energy and activity levels. They are equally at odds with available data when they assert "stress" associated with hard work, hot climates, high altitudes or injury boosts protein needs. They outdo themselves when they claim carbohydrates cause obesity and high protein diets are the answer to weight problems. Not only is there no call for high protein intake, but high protein leads to rapid degeneration of our very bone structure; it raises the blood levels of nitrogenous waste products to dangerous levels, and it brings a debilitating lack of endurance. If there is one period of life when it is believed that humans need a high level of protein it is during infancy yet human milk is lower in protein than even potatoes. Advocates of high protein intake could do no worse than defend so-called "protein foods," namely meat, eggs and dairy products: actually these products derive more than half their calories from fat, and the combination of animal protein and animal fat is the very essence of our problem.

It is the purpose of this book to demonstrate beyond a doubt that the degenerative diseases which plague the Western world today are a direct result of our diet; and to show that there is an alternative which promises a state of health above any seen in recorded history.

There are many alternatives to normal diets, of course. Any vegetarian diet that is free of salt and processed foods is bound to be an improvement over normal diets. Most whole-foods, strict vegetarian diets require nothing more than a source of vitamin B_{12} to be sound nutritionally. But having come from the worst diet ever known we are prepared to seek the best diet ever eaten. It is actually very simple to construct a diet better than any recorded. A diet based on raw sprouts and raw, dark-green leaf vegetables with a little seaweed or other algae (referred to as the SGA diet) provides maximal amounts of what humans need and avoids the substances and practices that cause degeneration. The SGA diet needs only a source of additional calories which tubers or fruit can provide. It is simple to the point of requiring less land and resources than anything previously envisioned by researchers concerned with the future of the world.

A world with several times today's population could easily be fed with SGA-type diets. And it could be accomplished without the heavy use of resource-depleting and harmful farm chemicals and equipment. In the long run we must stem population growth, of course, and there is evidence we could also expect this with simple SGA-type diets. A close look at the world today shows simple, whole-foods, nutritionally complete vegetarian diets are the mark of not only long life and abounding health, but natural birth control in the form of constraint. The pill and abortions are increasing the severity of our sickness. Reliance on pills and surgery has brought us to the brink of total debilitation, and it is time to say "no thank you" to easy answers and the flow of convenience items that have robbed us of any semblance of individuality and freedom.

I spent three wonderful years at the Science and Invention Library of the British Museum in London and at the science libraries of the University of Texas in Austin trying to unravel the truth about what we are eating. The research required reviewing many thousands of research reports, and in time it became clear that one need not rely on the claims of food reformers to see the horrors of our diet. There is ample information in the reports appearing in the most respected technical journals, textbooks and other publications to put an end to any defense of current eating practices. The original transcript of this book carried well over 2000 references and was written for those with a working knowledge of nutrition, degenerative disease and statistics. At the suggestion of my publisher, however, the transcript was rewritten so that there are now no training prerequisites. The number of references were reduced and references were annotated by paragraph at the end of the book in an effort to facilitate reading by avoiding distracting footnotes. For those who wish to pursue further verification for the claims in this book, the notes are there and provide strong substantiation for every major claim.

Perhaps this will be, as my publisher believes, a brick added to the structure of change. But it is my sincere belief that every time someone moves in the direction of simplicity in his or her diet and life-style a brick is added to that structure. If there is a better way of eating than an SGA-type of diet, we shall certainly discover it as long as we follow a way of simplicity while offering an open mind to all sources of knowledge.

1 / cancer

Cells belonging to the same organ, gland or structural component of the body are, as a rule metabolically similar and specialized in that they synthesize only those proteins which are necessary for the functioning of the structure they compose. For example, liver cells tend to specialize in the production of proteins used as catalysts (enzymes) for liver functions and muscle cells specialize in the production of muscle proteins.[1]

In cancer, cells lose their specialized protein producing capacities and all malignant cells tend to function the same regardless of where they occur in the body. The normal mechanisms which stop excess protein synthesis and cell multiplication seem to be lost. Malignant cells tend to accumulate protein until cell division is forced, and since the aberrant cells lack the ability to produce speific proteins they become in effect growth specialists.[2]

Protein synthesis is accelerated by increased protein intake so it is reasonable to suspect cancer may be related to an excess of dietary protein. Actually cancer bears a close tie to not only excess protein but growth promoters of all kinds, including high caloric intake, high fat levels, overproduction of sex hormones and high intake of growth promoting vitamins. Obese individuals, women with big breasts and individuals who take an excess of calories, a high level of fat or large amounts of meat have all been singled out as high risk cases in a number of the most widespread cancers.[3]

Growth promoting diets predate recorded history . . . and so does cancer. Tumors have been found in Neolithic bones, in Egyptian mummies and in the bones of pre-Columbian American Indians. Greek medical literature has many references to malignant tumors and Galen, writing during the second century, A.D., had hundreds of passages on cancer, indicating the disease was not uncommon in surfeit Rome.[4]

Over the last two centuries cancer treatment has been a source of
ceaseless controversy between dissident practitioners and medical officialdom. Mild vegetarian diets designed to give a rest to the body,
especially the liver, have been used by numerous dissidents but advocates of gruesome conventional treatments refused, until quite recently, to acknowledge a strong relationship between cancer and
dietary excesses. All the while there were dissidents who seemed to
have considerable success in treating cancer. Dr. Max Gerson, a
German physician who immigrated to New York when Hitler came
to power, treated cancer with a diet of selected fruits and vegetables
and told a Senate subcommittee that "beginning cancers are easy to
treat." He estimated only about 30% of "the most hopeless cases"
responded favorably to his treatment. Gerson strongly believed the
root cause of the cancer problem was the Western diet and that an
overhaul of the diet would bring an end to the disease. Groups taking
whole foods—mostly vegetarian diets—do tend to avoid cancer.[5]

Dr. W. A. Price crossed five continents finding no evidence of
cancer among members of isolated self-sufficient societies. An American doctor who spent a major portion of his life in isolated regions
of Brazil and Ecuador reported not a single case of cancer among the
60,000 inhabitants of those areas. The renowned anthropologist, Dr.
Sula Benet, reports the many researchers observing the rural
Abkhasians (USSR) have yet to discover a case of cancer and an
eminent British physician who spent ten years among the de facto
vegetarian Hunzas said he "never saw a case" of cancer. Dr. Albert
Schweitzer said "where there is no civilization there is no cancer,"
adding that both the Hunzas and Ethiopians had remained free of the
disease.[6]

(It will be good to note here that throughout this book frequent
references will be made to the Abkhasians who live on the Black Sea
in the USSR, the Hunzas who live in the Himalayas of Northern Pakistan and the Vilcabambas who reside in the Andes of Ecuador. Each
of these three groups have been rigorously observed and studied by
the medical and scientific worlds because of their remarkable good
health and longevity. As will be demonstrated during the course of
this book these groups partake of diets which are principally vegetarian.)[7]

Differences in cancer incidence and mortality rates support the association between civilization and cancer. The cancer death rate among West German males is fifteen times the rate for males in El Salvador. Adjusted for age differences the West German rate is still six times as high. The age adjusted incidence of cancer for whites in Laredo, Texas is twice as high as the incidence for Mexican-Americans in the same city. The Seventh Day Adventists, only about half of whom are vegetarian, have a much lower cancer mortality rate than Americans as a whole. Exhibit C1 lists some representative mortality rates while Exhibit C2 gives some related incidence rates.[8]

Exhibit C1

Cancer Mortality Rates (1964)

Country	Raw cancer death rate (per 100,000)		Age adjusted death rate (per 100,000)	
	MALES	FEMALES	MALES	FEMALES
Ceylon	24	22	24	25
Mexico	31	46	34	50
Yugoslavia	96	82	68	51
Portugal	115	105	72	56
United States	170	139	92	70
U.S. Seventh Day Adventists	100	90	55	45
Scotland	254	204	124	81

Sources: Preston, S.H. et al. "Causes of Death", Seminar Press, 1972; New York Post, June 24, 1974; Adventist Health Study, Loma Linda University, 1974.

Exhibit C2

Age adjusted cancer incidence rates
(cases per 100,000 population)

LOCALITY	MALES	FEMALES	COMBINED *
Ibadan, Nigeria	76.7	104.8	91
Israeli Arabs	132.2	70.7	96
Bombay	139.5	131.1	135
Rural Poland	165.2	131.1	148
Warsaw	214.9	204.7	210
Denmark	221.1	223.3	222
Birmingham England	254.5	196.3	225
Connecticut (whites)	257.8	220.0	239
Harlingen, Texas (whites)	452.6	353.5	403

*Simple average of males and females
Source: MacDonald, EJ. Cancer Bul. 25(2):33,1973.

It has been estimated that over 700,000 Americans will develop cancer during 1975. One fourth of those living in the U.S. today are expected to eventually acquire cancer. Thus chances are three to one that at least one member of a family of four will develop the disease. It's just about even odds at least one member of a family of four will die of cancer.[9]

To the surprise of many, white Americans were just about as susceptible to cancer 50 years ago as they are today. Studies by the National Cancer Institute (NCI) only go back to 1937, but the NCI data shows the age adjusted incidence of cancer among U.S. whites rose only 6% between 1937 and 1969. Without a sharp rise in lung cancer the incidence would have remained virtually unchanged. The data actually shows a decline for white females.[10]

Studies indicate that few induced cancers take less than 15 years to develop, therefore the high incidence of cancer among U.S. whites in 1937 indicates the factors leading to the alarmingly high incidence of the disease that year were in effect by 1922. But if this be the case, the root causes came prior to

* the widespread use of food additives,
* the extensive use of farm chemicals,
* radiation from fall out, x-ray, etc.,
* gross environmental pollution and
* high levels of stress and social disarray.[11]

Like cancer, these factors are hallmarks of a "high standard" of living but unlike cancer, they were not major problems during the 1920's. Obviously then, we must look beyond these factors to find a meaningful explanation of the long-standing high incidence of cancer among U.S. whites.[12]

The reason for focusing on whites is that blacks have experienced a marked increase in susceptibility to cancer in recent years. Government statistics show the incidence for black males rose from two-thirds the rate for whites in 1937 to a level above that for whites in 1969. The increase has been accompanied by substantial, if not radical, changes in eating habits, but this association is clouded by other changes.[13]

FOOD INTAKE AND OBESITY

With animals one of the surest ways to avoid becoming susceptible to cancer is to eat less. Dr. Albert Tannenbaum who pioneered in studies relating food intake and cancer, reported "at least eight different types of tumors and leukemia of the mouse are inhibited by caloric restriction. Furthermore, as yet, no tumor has been found that does not respond this way." He cited the favorable results of restricted food consumption on spontaneous breast tumors, induced skin tumors, lung cancer and leukemia.[14]

A renowned authority on the biochemistry of cancer, Dr. Jesse Greenstein, found caloric restrictions led to a drop in the incidence of breast cancer from 38% to zero in one strain of mice and from almost 100% to very low levels in another strain. A twenty-year study of beef cattle showed 14% of the heavy, large animals fed on prime pastures and given supplements developed spontaneous eye cancer. Only 1.5% of the cattle subjected to low-level feeding on poor pastures were afflicted.[15]

Dr. R. H. Ross and a colleague at the Institute for Cancer Research extended the study of the relationship between caloric intake and cancer incidence in animals to include tumors of the lymph system, connective tissue, endocrine glands and other sites. They found that the overall incidence of tumors was cut 90% by restricting the animals' intake throughout their lives. The life-span of the animals on a restricted intake was half again as long as that of those given free access to food, and the age adjusted incidence of tumors among those on lower intake was only one-twenty-fifth that of those given free access to food.[16]

Tannenbaum and an associate found the incidence of induced skin tumors in experimental animals was markedly reduced even when caloric restrictions were not begun until after lengthy exposure to a carcinogen (cancer causing agent). On the other hand, caloric restriction alone does not as a rule, lead to the disappearances of existing tumors in animals. If something more is needed to cure cancer in animals, cutting food intake goes a long way in preventing the disease. The same is true of humans.[17]

Excessive food intake, increasing body weight and obesity have all been related to an increase in the occurrence of cancer in humans. Ironically, insurance company mortality records which are usually used to support the association between obesity and cancer mortality, tend to greatly understate the case. Consider for example, the 50-

year-old report of the Union Central Life Insurance Company shown
in Exhibit C3. The report was derived from the records of 192,000
men who bought policies in Dublin at age 45 or beyond and who
were classified by weight at issuance of policy.[18]

Exhibit C3

Cancer mortality rates for various weight classes
of Union Central Life Insurance Company policyholders who were issued coverage
after age 45 in Dublin between 1880 and 1920.

WEIGHT AT ISSUANCE OF POLICY	CANCER DEATH RATE PER 100,000
25% or more overweight	143
15–25% overweight	138
5–15% overweight	121
Normal weight	111
5–15% underweight	114
15–50% underweight	95

The Union Central figures fail to take into account the longer life
of thinner men. Added years mean not only added exposure to cancer,
but exposure during high-risk advanced years. Exhibit C4 shows how
rapidly the cancer death rate advanced with age during the time of the
Dublin study.[19]

Exhibit C4

Cancer mortality rate for U.S. men in 1900

AGE	CANCER DEATHS PER 100,000
47.5	56
57.5	140
67.5	350
77.5	490
87.5	520

Source: Preston, S.H., et al. "Causes of Death," p. 724, Seminar Press, 1972.

It is not difficult to estimate the average life expectancy of men of
any given age beyond 45 in Dublin during 1880–1920. Life expectancy at any age greater than 40 varies little by nationality or with
time. The expected age of death of Union Central's policyholders
who were issued policies at ages 47 and 55 are given in Exhibit C5.
The figures given for those above or below normal weight are based
on adjustments suggested by Ross and others. Using these and other
data, it is possible to estimate the cancer mortality rates for the Union

Central policyholders as a function of both age and weight class. (*See Appendix 3 for detailed analysis*).[20]

Exhibit C5

Expected age of death of men in Dublin from 1880–1920.

Expected age at time of death

AGE	20% UNDERWEIGHT	NORMAL WEIGHT	25% OVERWEIGHT
47	77	71.5	62
55	78	73	66

Exhibit C6 translates the insurance data into mortality rates for U.S. men in 1969. It indicates the cancer mortality rate for 40-year-old men 25% overweight is 370 per 100,000 compared to 101 per 100,000 for 40-year-olds who are 20% below the average weight. By the time these thin men reach age 52, however, their cancer mortality rate would have risen to the rate of obese men of age 40. Perhaps this explains why so little attention is given to the relationship between obesity and cancer. But it does not justify this lack of attention for results like these may be important links in a chain of observations which form a plan for preventing cancer. It is interesting that the rural Abkhasians, who live much longer than Americans, and yet give no evidence of cancer, regard overeating as dangerous and consider obesity an illness. They remain "slim, but strong" reports Benet.[21]

Exhibit C6

Estimated incidence of cancer for U.S. males in 1969

	Deaths per 100,000	
WEIGHT CLASS	AGE 40	AGE 52
25% overweight	370	1320
Normal	140	500
20% underweight	101	360

Obese women, like their male counterparts, show a strong predisposition to cancer. Obesity will be discussed in some detail in Chapter 3 but it is well to state here that research with animals has shown growth-promoting diets, that is diets high in protein and fat, lead to gross obesity. The weights of rats and mice are often doubled by high intake of fat and protein. Obesity is associated with sharp reductions in physical activity and high fat, high protein diets may reduce activity by lowering endurance. Humans fed diets low in fat and protein have increased endurance and show sharp reductions in weight.[22]

Eating fewer times each day might lead to reduced intake. Numerous studies show animals that are "meal-fed," that is offered food only for a restricted time period (normally two hours) each day, consume considerably less food than animals given unlimited access to food. In most cases the meal-fed animals weigh less as well. It may be necessary to combine reduced fat intake with fewer meals to achieve a lower caloric intake, however. Animals do not adapt to meal-feeding when their fat intake is high.[23]

Eliminating processed foods from the diet should be an aid in preventing obesity. A fair proportion of rats fed highly processed foods become obese. Sugar may be the most undesirable processed carbohydrate: animals fed sugar tend to eat more and gain more weight than starch-fed animals.[24]

Normal American and European diets are very high in fat and protein and are dominated by processed foods, including sugar. Moreover, those who eat such diets seem to feel an almost incessant need for food and drink (as snacks, etc.). It is not surprising then that obesity is rampant in the industrialized West.[25]

High levels of dietary fat, protein and refined foods, especially sugar, have all been implicated directly in cancer in animals and humans. Thus a well-planned attack on obesity promises both direct and indirect defense against cancer.[26]

Vegetarian diets, which are usually relatively low in fat and protein result in considerably lower weight levels on the average. Especially effective are whole-foods vegan (strict vegetarians) diets which have led to rapid losses of weight to levels 10% to 20% under normal. Obesity is not seen among vegans who avoid processed foods and growth promoting supplements and take only limited amounts of oil-rich nuts and seeds. The SGA diet which is (*see Appendix 1 for a detailed description*) a mix of raw soy sprouts, other sprouts, raw dark green leaf vegetables and tubers with a little seaweed, has all the attributes of the most effective weight control diets and has resulted in troublefree transitions from obesity to slimness.[27]

Obesity has been linked to various degenerative processes and is usually accompanied by serious metabolic disorders. One study showed 94 of 100 obese children suffered from impaired liver function and obesity greatly increases the risk of cirrhosis of the liver. The liver may be the last, and most important, defense against cancer.[28]

THE LIVER

The livers of animals with cancer undergo changes in total solids, lipids, enzyme activity, vitamin content and mineral concentrations. Presumably, liver dysfunction precedes the appearance of cancer. When severe liver cirrhosis was induced in rats by a single dietary deficiency, all of the affected animals developed at least one tumor. Sites included the lungs, pancreas, bladder and liver itself.[29]

The liver seems no less involved in human cancer. Cancer researchers found every one of 50 patients suffering from cancers of the gastrointestinal tract had at least one liver dysfunction. Most had four or more. The livers of most members of a comparable group without cancer evidenced no liver disorder, and the livers of patients whose tumors had been removed by surgery showed some improvement. Experts point to regeneration of the liver as a basic concern of cancer researchers, and Greenstein concluded there is "little doubt that hepatic (liver) insufficiency is a concomitant phenomenon with cancer."[30]

The normal human liver allegedly produces a substance which powerfully inhibits the growth of tumors in animals. The factor, called TIP (Tumor Inhibitory Principle) is not found in the livers of cancer patients but the discoverer of TIP, Dr. John G. Kidd of Cornell, and others have found TIP-like activity in liver extracts of cancer-free hogs, rabbits, horses, cows, sheep and humans. Administration of liver extracts resulted in the disappearance of a number of tumors in mice with breast tumors and cut by two-thirds the incidence of tumors in another group of animals. An extract of yeast which yielded dramatic reductions in animal tumors is believed to enhance the "natural defenses" of the animals, possibly by stimulating the production of TIP.[31]

Acupuncturists use a delicate system of "taking pulses" to judge the condition of the internal organs of patients. The head of the famous Branksome Acupuncture Clinic in Kenilworth, England, Dr. John D'Ambrosio says cancer patients invaribly suffer from liver malfunction and that the success of the acupuncturist's treatment depends on his or her ability to revitalize the liver. The highly successful American physician, Dr. Henry Bieler who used simple vegetarian diets to treat all manners of illness, claims that when the liver fails to deal with toxins, cancer can occur, and Gerson reasoned "the liver is the center of the restoration process in those cancer patients who improve strikingly. If the liver is too far destroyed then the treatment cannot be effective."[32]

It has been clearly demonstrated that liver damage, thence cancer, can be induced by diet and Ross reports liver activity in rats is "significantly influenced" by diet. Ross' variables were restricted to carbohydrate, fat and protein with each of these variables alternating in predominance in a diet mix.[33]

Alcohol, a carbohydrate, can severely damage the livers of rats, especially in the presence of a high fat diet. Even with so-called "adequate" diets, that is diets supplemented with vitamins and minerals, alcohol-fed baboons developed fatty livers. In a long term study of hospital records in Boston, it was found chronic alcoholism was involved in more than half of all deaths due to liver cancer. Alcohol has been implicated in other cancers also. Per capita consumption of alcohol in the U.S. rose steadily from 1860 till 1920, and it seems safe to assume cancer was on the rise throughout this period. Both alcohol intake and cancer leveled off after 1920.[34]

Sugar is another carbohydrate which can damage the liver. Sugar tends to cause an accumulation of fat in the livers of rats, and the condition is made worse by even small amounts of cooked egg. The liver tissue of normal humans showed pathological changes when their sugar intake was raised.[35]

The adverse effects of sugar on the liver are not likely to be avoided by supplements. Animals are usually provided with a complete array of vitamins and minerals when the effects of sugar are examined. It has been suggested that sugar may raise the need for choline, but two researchers found the livers of rats fed sugar plus choline contained twice as much fat as the livers of rats fed heated starch from which most of the choline had been removed. It has been suggested supplemental chromium might offset the effect of sugar on the liver but tests showed chromium supplements did not prevent sugar from elevating liver lipids.[36]

When rats were given a powerful carcinogen (cancer promoting substance) in a diet containing semi-synthetic cooked starch, 19% of the animals developed skin tumors. When a simple sugar was substituted for the starch, however, the tumor incidence rose by 60%. It has been shown in other experiments that highly processed foods raise the incidence of spontaneous liver tumors and induced tumors of the digestive tract in rats. Quite possibly, it is through the effect of refined foods on the liver that such foods boost the incidence of cancer.[37]

Per capita consumption of simple sugars in the U.S. was a very high 90 grams per day in 1900 and reached current levels in the early 20's. The same is true of the incidence of cancer and it is claimed that isolated groups remained free of cancer until sugar and refined flour were added to their diets. Neither the Hunzas nor the Abkhasians take any sugar. The Abkhasians do use a little honey, however.[38]

Cola drinks and "regular" coffee may offer double taxation to the liver. These common crutches contain not only sugar, but caffeine, which is believed to cause fatty build-ups in the livers of humans. Caffeine is a required constituent of cola drinks. Coffee may affect lipid disorders even after the caffeine has been removed, and coffee has been implicated directly in cancers of the kidney, bladder and female sex organs.[39]

High protein intake, particularly in the presence of pyridoxine (vitamin B6) deficiency, can cause fatty livers and two components of meat and eggs, cholesterol and cholic acid, led to fatty degeneration of the livers of hamsters and mice in only one month. Feeding normal and diabetic rats cholesterol with different fats led to fatty livers in just six weeks. A build-up of liver fat was more pronounced in the diabetic animals but all groups showed evidence of fatty cirrhosis. The cholesterol-fed animals also experienced an increase in liver cholesterol. In a study at Auburn University it was found supplemental choline did not prevent build-ups in liver cholesterol in rats fed cholesterol and beef fat. In an unrelated study it was found that cholesterol alone caused marked increases in the liver cholesterol of germ-free rats. Only animal foods contain cholesterol, and there is evidence that cholesterol-rich eggs can injure the liver.[40]

Diets containing fresh eggs, dried whole egg, or raw egg and de-fatted egg powder have all resulted in high concentrations of fat and cholesterol in the livers of rats. Gerson reported he lost three cancer patients when he let them take half an egg yolk per day, and the founder of a cancer treatment clinic in Texas claimed most cancer patients were heavy egg eaters. [41]

A class of fat found in meat and eggs caused a defect in rabbits, suggestive of severe liver dysfunction. Studies have shown high fat intake can cause deranged carbohydrate metabolism in the livers of rats, and an Indian physician found most patients with impaired carbohydrate metabolism responded very favorably to low-fat, sugar-free diets. [42]

The kidneys and livers of mice became enlarged after 108 days on lean ground meat, and when cholesterol-containing fractions of various animal products including pigs liver, cow's milk and human liver were injected into mice, they caused tumors in a substantial number of the animals. [43]

In the past the Eskimos are alleged to have remained free of cancer in spite of a flesh-rich diet but they took their flesh raw, much of their flesh was from fish and when they did eat mammalian flesh, they ate all of the internal organs as well. And they ate no eggs. Nor do the cancer-free Hunzas eat eggs; the Abkahasians occasionally eat eggs and meat but neither constitutes a significant part of their diet. Meat and/or animal protein have been implicated directly in breast cancer, cancer of the bowel and pancreatic cancer. It is interesting to note that the intake of meat and eggs in the U.S. was already near current levels by 1919. [44]

It appears then, that the liver is vital to the body's defense against cancer and the integrity of the liver is strongly influenced by the diet. The liver may be damaged by vitamin deficiencies, an excess of protein without a substantial increase in vitamin B6 or simply excesses of calories, alcohol, sugar, eggs, meat, refined grains or fats. Fresh fruits and vegetable juices have been used to treat damaged livers. However, a diet high in soybean sprouts, grain sprouts, bean sprouts and green leaf vegetables is apt to yield more lasting results: sprouts and greens are much richer than fruits and other vegetables in a broad spectrum of nutrients (including vitamin B6) that are required by the liver. At the same time, sprouts and greens are low in fat and calories, contain no cholesterol, need no cooking or refining and are not excessive in protein.[45]

DIETARY LIPIDS

While dietary fat has been implicated in cancer via its role in obesity and liver impairment, direct links between fat and cancer are strong and growing. Laboratory studies have implicated various fats in the development of tumors in animals and high levels of total fats, animal fats and other lipids, including cholesterol, have been associated with numerous cancers in humans. It was once thought leukemia might be unresponsive to dietary fat but it was recently found rats on an "adequate" diet containing 20% chicken fat had a high incidence of leukemia. Fats can lower the body resistance to cancer, act as carcinogens themselves, serve as carriers for fat-related carcinogens or cause the body to produce excesses of substances, which, in sufficient quantity, may be carcinogenic.[46]

Rats fed a commercial dye all developed liver tumors on a diet containing 20% corn oil. High fat levels raise the rate of formation of spontaneous liver tumors and breast cancer in mice, and fats also facilitate an increase in carcinogen-induced breast cancer in female rats. Gerson said recessed tumors reappeared when patients were fed fats. Dr. M. W. Sterns, Jr., chief of colon-rectal service at the Sloan-Kittering Cancer Center advises bowel cancer patients to tell their children to eat less fat. High-fat intake has been linked to bowel cancer by a number of researchers, and a large scale study in New York linked breast cancer to several diet-related factors, including high-fat intake. The president of the American Cancer Society said recently that both breast cancer and cancer of the colon "are related to a high fat and animal protein diet." Dr. E. L. Wynder, president, American Health Foundation warns that high fat diets may be responsible for some cases of kidney and pancreatic cancers also. Fat intake is already implicated in more new cases of cancer each year than smoking. It behooves the American Cancer Society to complement its very commendable antismoking campaign with a program aimed at getting individuals to lower fat intake.[47]

Oleic acid, in which olive oil, animal fats and peanut oil are high, induced tumors in mice, rats and rabbits. The standard American diet contains about 50 grams of oleic acid per day, two-thirds of which is derived from meat, eggs, poultry and dairy products. The cancer-free Hunzas and Abkhasians take less than 15 grams of oleic acid per day.[48]

The first step in the digestion of fats is emulsification (separation into small droplets) which occurs in the intestines in the presence of liver bile. The amount of bile excreted depends on the amount of fat ingested and on the typical U.S. diet of 45% fat, individuals have much higher levels of bile entering their intestines than do Japanese, Ugandans or U.S. vegetarians. With an excess of bile goes an excess of bile acids and at least one bile acid, deoxycholic acid, gave rise to tumors in mice.[49]

Bile components can be altered by the bacteria in the intestines and deoxycholic acid may, in the presence of intestinal bacteria, be transformed into a so-called cyclic-hydrocarbon which is among the most carcinogenic substances known to man. Cyclic-hydrocarbons have been found to induce cancers of the connecting tissue, skin, lungs, stomach, intestines, brain and blood of various animals. If deoxycholic acid is not transformed into a carcinogenic cyclic-hydrocarbon, the most abundant bile acid, cholic acid, may be. The same cyclic-hydrocarbon that arises from deoxycholic acid can be produced from cholic acid by the same simple chemical changes which are always taking place in the intestines. Rats failed to develop tumors when exposed to pure bile acids, but when the bile acids were exposed to intestinal bacteria from a patient with cancer of the rectum the animals developed cancer themselves. It is believed that bile components may be involved in cancers of the stomach, breast, colon and rectum of humans.[50]

It might require dramatic reductions in fat intake on the part of individuals accustomed to normal American and European diets to achieve significant protection against cancer. Cancer has been induced in animals by diets containing considerably smaller proportions of fat than most Westerners consume. One researcher found cutting the fat intake of laboratory animals from levels in excess of the U.S. average to normal U.S. levels had little effect on the incidence of skin tumors. Tannenbaum found the incidence of breast tumors in mice fell when fat levels were cut to one-third of normal U.S. Levels and a further cut to less than 10% of normal U.S. fat intake doubled the reduction in tumors. It is not surprising there has been no significant change in the incidence of cancer during the anti-coronary studies. Such experiments have never been designed to cut fat levels under 28% of calories and the preference for peanut oil and corn oil over say, coconut oil, is at odds with cancer research findings. The Hunzas and Abkhasians take only a quarter to a third the amount of fat Americans normally consume.[51]

CHOLESTEROL

Cholesterol, which is contained in all animal foods and is both a fat-related substance and a bile component, may be directly involved in various cancers. Dietary cholesterol has led to liver derangements in rats, and mice developed tumors when injected with cholesterol-rich extracts from human livers. Cholesterol alone and cholesterol-rich extracts from cream and milk have also induced tumors in mice. There is a tendency for cholesterol to build up in the liver when dietary cholesterol is high, and impaired cholesterol metabolism by the liver is common in human cancers.[52]

In liver cancer, the malignant cells are unable to use dietary cholesterol for the synthesis of bile acids and the cholesterol synthesized by the malignant tissue is released into the bloodstream. The synthesis of cholesterol and related compounds is elevated tenfold in leukemia in mice and the uncontrolled oxidation of cholesterol is a feature of cancer of the adrenal cortex. Impaired cholesterol synthesis is common in cancer of the gastrointestinal tract also.[53]

Enlarged prostate glands, which presumably precede cancer of the prostate, are enhanced by relatively high output of androgens (male sex hormones). Androgens are synthesized from cholesterol: animal products, all of which contain cholesterol tend to promote androgen production.[54]

Gall bladder cancer is almost always preceded by gallstones and dietary cholesterol leads rapidly to gallstones in laboratory animals: prairie dogs fed 1.2% cholesterol had gallstones in only 14 days. Autopsies showed about 11% of U.S. females and 7% U.S. males had gallstones. More than two thirds of the U.S. gallstones consisted primarily of cholesterol. Gallstones were far less common and less frequently formed from cholesterol among Japanese who take much less dietary cholesterol and fat than Americans.[55]

Even when the liver transforms dietary cholesterol into bile acids, rather than allowing cholesterol to build up in the liver tissue, the danger of cancer is not ended. Both bile acids and cholesterol may be altered by intestinal bacteria to form carcinogens which induce cancer of the bowel. Cancer of the bowel (colon and rectum) is the most prevalent cancer in America, and it has been associated with intake of meat, especially beef, eggs and animal fat, all of which are high in cholesterol. There is a negative correlation between cancer of the colon and (cholesterol free) cereal intake.[56]

The second most prevalent cancer in the U.S. is breast cancer and meat, eggs and fat have been implicated in breast cancer also. Whether the cholesterol in animal products plays a role in breast cancer is unknown.[57]

One of the fastest rising cancers is cancer of the pancreas which has been associated with high intake of meat and a high intake of meat combined with a low intake of vegetables in Japan. A close association between the incidence of pancreatic cancer and dietary fat is supported by an association between prior diabetes and cancer of the pancreas in women. But animal fat contains cholesterol, and there is a correlation between pancreatic cancer and gall bladder disease in which cholesterol is strongly implicated.[58]

The degree of involvement of dietary cholesterol in cancer may be somewhat academic since cholesterol-bearing (i.e. animal) products have been strongly implicated in most of the major cancers. On the other hand, heated cholesterol may pose a special problem. When cholesterol was heated to 360°C it yielded a mix of seven products, six of which are intermediates in the transformation into the same highly carcinogenic cyclic-hydrocarbon that may arise from the bile acids. Greenstein concluded that the possibility that the cancer causing substance might be formed by heating cholesterol "cannot be excluded."[59]

The cholesterol in oil dripping from steaks during charcoal broiling can become superheated and render the meat highly carcinogenic. It was reported that a single charcoal broiled steak had as much cancer causing potency as a dozen packs of cigarettes.[60]

The observation that the Eskimos ate their prey raw takes added significance with the knowledge heated cholesterol may be considerably more carcinogenic than unheated cholesterol. The Hunzas and Abkhasians take little cholesterol and almost none that has been heated above 200°C. Evidently Americans have a daily intake of about 500 milligrams of cholesterol which has been subjected to cooking. That's up only slightly from an estimated 430 milligrams per day in 1910 which could be related to the high incidence of cancer in 1920.[61]

HYPERCALCEMIA

Among the metabolic disorders receiving increasing attention from cancer researchers is hypercalcemia (high blood calcium). Hypercalcemia has been found to be common in cases of lung cancer, breast cancer, cancer of the kidney, leukemia, tumors of the head, neck and esophagus and other cancers. Hypercalcemia could result from excessive calcium intake but it more likely results from an overactive parathyroid gland or other disorders associated with increased bone resorption (that is loss of bone structure by the bones being dissolved by the blood).[62]

Bone resorption has been linked to high protein intake in humans and high phosphorus intake in animals and humans. It also results from inactivity in humans. Two scientists who studied the relationship between high phosphorus intake and bone resorption extensively claim the high intake of meat, eggs, fish and beans in the U.S. is responsible for a low calcium to phosphorus ratio of the U.S. diet. These same foods, along with dairy products, add to the risk of resorption of bone calcium by their high protein content. A diet high in meat led to bone resorption at rates two-to-three times the rates of bone growth in rats and the meat-eating humans seem to suffer an analogous fate. A comparative study of vegetarians and meat-eaters indicated meat-eating women had lower bone densities than vegetarian women.[63]

If vegetarians are the best protected group against hypercalcemia, many "health food" advocates are likely to be the most vulnerable. Excesses of vitamin A, phosphorus and protein all of which are popular among those who believe malnutrition is a matter of deficiencies can all raise blood calcium. Gerson said giving a calcium compound to youths suffering from bone tumors brought on incurable regrowths.[64]

PROTEIN

Cancerous cells, it may be recalled, are characterized by excessive protein synthesis and since increasing protein intake accelerates protein synthesis, high protein intake must be regarded as a threat in cancer. All of the dietary treatments for cancer which achieved acclaim were and are low in protein and even orthodox medical practitioners are being forced to cast a critical eye at high protein intake.[65]

It has been known for some time that animals taking low-protein diets often show decreases in the incidence, growth and spread of tumors. Ross and a colleague undertook massive studies to clarify the interrelationships between protein intake, calories and the incidence of spontaneous tumors in male rats. They found protein intake had little influence on the very high incidence of tumors in animals fed an unlimited amount of food but reducing the protein intake of rats on a restricted calorie regime resulted in cutting the incidence of tumors almost in half. However, Ross' experiments may have greatly underestimated the value of low protein intake for the low-protein diet used was more than two thirds sugar while the high protein ratio contained a relatively small amount of sugar. As pointed out, sugar has been implicated in liver damage, impaired carbohydrate metabolism and the increased incidence of cancer in animals.[66]

Another researcher found that when mice were fed a low protein diet, implanted tumors grew very slowly and a number of tumors actually disappeared. He concluded a "low-protein diet favors natural body defences" against cancer. Other animal studies suggest the effect of protein levels may be greater for certain types of cancer than others.[67]

High intake of protein, especially animal proteins, has been implicated in the leading female cancers, bowel cancer which is the leading cancer affecting both sexes and cancer of the pancreas which is possibly the most rapidly rising form of cancer in the U.S. Animal proteins are high in the amino acid lysine along with the sulfur-containing amino acids, and animals show increased resistance to cancer when fed proteins low in those amino acids. Bieler treated his first cancer patient with a diet low in the sulfur containing amino acids. Previously his patient had been taking a great deal of chicken but with Bieler's "sulfur-free" vegetarian diet the patient's tumor slowly disappeared.[68]

The primary reason for holding protein suspect in cancer is its ability to enhance rapid growth. In addition, excess protein is strongly implicated in human obesity, liver damage and hypercalcemia which greatly widens its possible role in cancer. The Hunzas take about half as much protein as Americans while the Abkhasians take about 25% less than the U.S. on the average. Just what constitutes an excess of protein depends a great deal on total caloric intake, however. The much lower caloric intake of the Abkhasians renders their protein needs much higher than that of Americans. The same is true of low-fat vegetarian diets. The basic SGA diet, for example, derives a very high percentage of total calories from protein; but caloric intake from the basic SGA diet is, of necessity, limited, so actual protein intake is never excessive. Moreover, low protein tubers and fruit are usually added to the SGA staples for calories so that the percentage of calories derived from protein declines as caloric intake increases. An increased caloric intake by individuals taking the standard U.S. diet is of itself very harmful and it invariably involves increases in protein, fat, or refined carbohydrates, all of which make the situation worse.[69]

VITAMINS AND MINERALS

The role of vitamins in cancer is complex. Deficiencies of some vitamins can weaken resistance if they threaten the integrity of the liver but excesses can weaken resistance if they promote rapid growth. There are studies indicating riboflavin deficiency reduces the incidence of tumors in animals and inhibits tumor growth in experimental animals and possibly in humans. Deficiencies in pantothenic acid and thiamin slowed tumor growth in animals but the animals experienced severe losses in body weight. Vitamin antagonists have been the focus of considerable effort in the field of chemotherapy.[70]

Folacin, or folic acid, in which sprouted beans and grains, green vegetables and raw liver are rich, resulted in the complete regression of tumors of 38 of 89 breast cancer-bearing mice. Folacin also inhibited the growth of transplanted tumors in mice. Vitamin C, in which green vegetables are very rich, apparently blocks the action of at least one carcinogen in the livers of rats. Another nutrient in which the U.S. diet is extremely low and in which sprouts and leaf vegetables are rich is manganese, and it has been hypothesized that manganese deficiency may trigger metabolic changes resulting in human cancer.[71]

It was recently discovered that gastrointestinal cancer patients had significantly lower levels of selenium in their blood than normal. Low serum selenium was seen with Hodgkin's disease, hepatitis, and liver cirrhosis also. An adequate selenium intake reduces tumor formation in animals and so-called antioxidants (including selenium, vitamin C and vitamin E) protected tissue cultures from damage by carcinogens. It is claimed that a significantly lower cancer mortality rate was found in areas where selenium intake is high. Whole grains are evidently the richest source of utilizable selenium and green leafy vegetables are extremely rich in the antioxidants, vitamins E and C. The standard U.S. diet is low in selenium and vitamin E and many persons may be taking little vitamin C.[72]

Molybdenum deficiency is suspected of playing a role in cancer of the esophagus. Lack of molybdenum may lead to the formation of a class of cancer causing substances known as nitrosamines. Beans and peas are evidently much higher in molybdenum than other foods but green leafy vegetables are good sources of the mineral also. The U.S. diet tends to be very low in molybdenum. Since a mix of sprouts and green leafy vegetables is high in all of the vitamins and minerals mentioned, it should provide a considerable degree of defense against cancer.[73]

One of the more interesting substances that has been employed in treating cancer is a substance known as laetrile or vitamin B17. Evidently, cancerous tissues accumulate an enormous excess of a group of enzymes which have the capacity to free cyanide from laetrile. Free cyanide can be detoxified by an enzyme found in normal cells but lacking in malignant cells so that cancer tissue has no defense against cyanide. Thus it would be hoped that administering laetrile to cancer patients should cause selective destruction of cancer cells without harming healthy tissue. Laetrile seems to have reversed a number of cancers and it is said to give "even better results" when the liver function can be improved: the liver must deal with toxic elements released from the malignant lesion. Laetrile is said to yield no side effects. It is found in many edible plants but animal products apparently contain little or none. Grasses, millet and seeds from fruits and vegetables are believed to be excellent sources of laetrile. It is important to know that the laetrile content of lentils, mungbeans and alfalfa is increased fiftyfold with sprouting. The extent to which laetrile contributes to the preventive capacities of plant foods is unknown, but raw sprouts, vegetables and fruits afford strong protection against cancer.[74]

Gerson, Bieler, the renowned naturopath C. Leslie Thomson, and others who have used diets to treat cancer have used "salt free" vegetarian diets. Gerson and Bieler placed strong emphasis on the need to give up the use of salt and Schweitzer connected the "increase of cancer with increased use of salt" in Africa. A portion of a group of animals injected with a saline solution developed cancer. During their era of immunity to cancer, the Eskimos used no salt, the cancer-free Abkhasians use little or no salt and the long-living Vilcabambas use no salt whatsoever. There is no question that high salt intake can adversely affect the health of animals and man.[75]

CANCER INCIDENCE VS. DIET

It should be clear that diet affects man's susceptibility to cancer profoundly. After stating categorically that half of all female cancers and almost a third of all male cancers can be related to diet, Wynder made it clear he was "not talking about food additives or cyclamates but about deficiencies and excesses in the regular diet." Wynder's assessment, shocking though it is, tends to be limited by the scope of past studies and does not allow for a possible relationship between diet and smoking. But more importantly it is tempered with limits on what dietary changes he regarded as possible and particularly to what extent calories might be cut or intake of animal products reduced. Dr. Fredrick Hoffman, who served as chief statistician for the Prudential Life Insurance Company, said "dietary influences are to be looked on as a causative factor in cancer." These influences include the quality of the raw foods collected, the nature and amount of processing used and the manner of preparation.[76]

By assigning relative values to these factors for the diets of various groups it is possible to derive cancer resistance ratings for each diet. By then correlating these ratings to cancer mortality or incidence rates it is then possible to make a reasoned guess at what sort of diet is necessary to prevent cancer and to predict the cancer mortality rate for any group on the basis of its dietary practices. The reader will be spared the mathematics but it is useful to review what led to specific ratings for quality processing and preparation. (*For those who wish to study the equation see Appendix 3.*)[77]

Whole grains, beans, vegetables, especially green leafy ones, should offer strong defense against cancer. They are rich in liver protecting vitamins, minerals and starch, free from cholesterol and bile acids, high in essential minerals, low in sugar and total fat as well as special fats implicated in cancer, and they do not promote rapid growth and large body size. In contrast, eggs and meat may weaken the liver, they are high in cholesterol, lack adequate amounts of key nutrients, are high in fat and oleic acid, tend to promote rapid growth and large body size and threaten to bring on hypercalcemia through bone resorption. Fruits, nuts, seafood, dairy products and oil seeds have some attributes plus some highly unfavorable characteristics. Salt, coffee beans, tea leaves, spices, etc. presumably contribute nothing to the body defenses and may even enhance the onset of cancer.[78]

Processing: Sprouting gets highest rating since it leads to enormous increases in vitamin content of whole grains and beans, lowers the fat content of seeds and rids beans of most of their phytic acid, and in doing so, raises the availability of a number of minerals. Conventional processing procedures tend to transform the most protective foods into threats to the body defenses. Grains are fermented to produce alcoholic beverages and sacrificed for the production of oil or nutritionally naked shadows of themselves such as white rice, commercial flour, degerminated corn, etc. Fruits are used for wine while cane and beets are transformed into that insidious symbol of kindness, sugar. Milk, seeds and legumes are often stripped of their oil; eggs, fruit, fish and milk can be dried or otherwise devitalized.[79]

Preparation: Highest rating goes to those who eat raw foods. Cooking destroys major portions of most of the B-complex along with other key nutrients. Cooking can degrade protein, oil and even carbohydrates. Heat adversely affects cholesterol, hence meat, eggs, fish, fowl and dairy products. Cooking can render the most protective foods impotent and may make animal foods carcinogenic.[80]

Quantity was not included as a factor in rating diets because of a strong correlation of reduced caloric intake with quality and lack of processing. The mathematics indicate a diet of whole grains, dairy products, fruit and vegetables with little cooking and little processing outside of a little cheesemaking should be more than adequate in preventing cancer. Thus, a cancer-preventing diet might include modest amounts of cooking oil, and even some flesh products on occasion.[81]

The mathematics also show that male adults who eat meat, fats, drink beer, eat sugar and white bread, etc. can expect a cancer incidence of 320 to 360 cases per 100,000. Now if such individuals set out to reduce their weight by eliminating eggs, fatty meats, butter, alcohol, sugar, cutting way back on visible fats and started to eat twice a day, one hour at each sitting, the incidence of cancer associated with their new diet would fall by 60% or more. Their diet would put them along side Nigerians, East Indians and gentiles in Israel, in terms of expected incidence of cancer, and judging by the appearance of these groups, our male adults could expect not only to lower the risk of cancer but to lower their weight as well.[82]

One interesting use of diet vs. incidence data is to estimate the total number of cancers we could expect if all the world began to eat like Westerners consuming large quantities of meat, sugar, refined grains, salt, coffee, alcohol and visible fats. With such a change we could expect more than 11,500,000 new cases of cancer each year with over 2,000,000 new cases per year in China alone. On the other hand, if all the world began to eat like the rural, inland Chinese we could expect no new cancer cases.[83]

Before tying together what has been said concerning cancer in general, it will be useful to make some observations about the more common types of cancer in the U.S. Women have some unique problems with respect to the sites of tumors.[84]

DISTINCTLY FEMALE CANCERS

Almost half of the female cancers recorded occur at sites associated with reproduction. The leading female cancers are listed below:

Site	Percent of Female Cancers	Total No. of New Cases Per Yr.
Breast	24%	78,000
Cervical Uteri	10%	34,000
Corpus Uteri	7%	24,000
Ovary	5%	16,000
Vulva and Vagina	1%	3,000
Total	47%	155,000

These malignancies are related to the inability of American women to render trouble-free birth and nourishment to children. There are also ties between "female" cancers and large, if stylish, breasts, early sex and promiscuity.[85]

Cancer of the breast is rare among women who nurse their own children. It occurs most frequently with unmarried women and married women who have no children or marry at a late age. Obesity raises the risk of breast cancer substantially.[86]

Cancer of the cervix (neck) of the uterus is most common in women who have sustained injury to the cervix during childbirth. It is also associated with promiscuity. The incidence of cervical cancer in women who began intercourse before age 17 is two to three times normal and the rate is higher in women who have had more than one partner. In contrast to cervical cancer, cancer of the corpus uteri usually occurs in women who have borne no children. Cancer of the corpus uteri is also associated with obesity, high blood pressure and disturbed carbohydrate metabolism.[87]

The capacity to reproduce and to breast feed one's offspring are indicators of general well-being. The former may be especially sensitive to factors implicated in cancer in general: high protein intake, obesity and over-cooking. It was found that as the protein intake of rats increased, the number of young produced decreased. It is claimed that reduced food intake raises productive capacity while obesity promotes sterility. Certainly on a worldwide basis high birth rates are associated with low-calorie, low-protein diets, low birth rates with the opposite.[88]

High caloric and protein intake leads to increased production of estrogens (female sex hormones) which in turn tends to promote various female cancers. High output of estrogens is necessary for the development of large breasts: less developed breasts do not yield to breast cancer in animals and large breasts greatly increase the risk of breast cancer in humans. Autopsies of 200 women who died of breast cancer showed evidence of prolonged overproduction of estrogens and excessive estrogen output has also been implicated in cancer of the uterus. Cancers of the uteri and ovary can be both induced in animals by estrogen.administration and researchers are now attempting to reverse the course of female cancers by hormone manipulation to reduce circulating estrogens. A safer approach would be simply to reduce food intake.[89]

Greenstein recognized high-calorie diets raised the incidence of breast tumors in laboratory animals by boosting estrogen output but he thought it might be necessary to reduce the caloric intake by 50% to "effectively prevent the appearance of tumors" and he feared this might abolish estrus and the capacity for bleeding. But others have found lesser reductions were capable of completely wiping out the appearance of breast tumors in mice, and Tannenbaum indicated food intake reductions of 30% to 40% were as effective as larger reductions. In any event, Ross' findings suggest cuts of 50% should improve the health of animals rather than impair it.[90]

A New York study showed high levels of dietary fat, obesity, large breasts and disturbed carbohydrate metabolism resulted in one and one-half to threefold increases in the risk of breast cancer. All of these factors are related to diet and estrogen production. With a "good model" for human breast cancer, it has been shown high fat promotes breast tumors in animals and the president of the American Cancer Society has openly admitted breast cancer is related to diets high in fat and animal protein. The relationships are backed not only by clinical studies but by statistical data from all over the world. In Japan, for example, intake of meat and dairy products is much lower than in the U.S., and Japanese women have an incidence of breast cancer only about one sixth that of American women. When Japanese immigrate to the U.S., however, their susceptibility to breast cancer rises markedly. Obesity, disturbed fat and carbohydrate metabolism and high blood pressure have all been implicated in cancer of the corpus uteri. Thus salt may play a role along with animal products, fats and refined foods, especially sugar, in cancer of the corpus uteri. Inadequate dietary folacin may also play a role in female cancers.[91]

Overall, it appears female cancers are very sensitive to caloric levels and growth-promoting fats and proteins. Salt, through its role in high blood pressure and sugar, through its ability to upset carbohydrate metabolism, may also be involved. Price said "a nonfunctional breast was unheard of" among the simple living groups he visited. Women who cut way down on animal products and saturated fats so as to restrain estrogen production, eliminate salt and sugar from the diet and do not habitually engage in sex with more than one partner are acting in accordance with findings which indicate low incidence of female cancers. They can further benefit by having natural childbirths and breast feeding their children. To these ends a simple, whole-foods, vegetarian diet should be ideal. While only half of the Seventh Day Adventists are believed to be vegetarian, Adventist women have mortality rates from female cancers 28% to 46% lower than non-Adventists.[92]

LUNG CANCER

The incidence of lung cancer in the United States has risen fivefold since 1937. The disease accounts for some 50,000 lives annually of which over 80% are men. There is considerable evidence that smoking contributes the principle carcinogenic activity in lung cancer and the inclination to smoke may be related to diet.[93]

Two physicians prepared slides from the lung tissue of 402 diseased males, 63 of whom died from lung cancer. Over 90% of the slides of light smokers and almost 100% of the slides of moderate smokers showed abnormalities; only 16.8% of the slides of nonsmokers revealed disturbances. Even more remarkable was their finding that 11% of the slides of the heavy smokers who had died of causes other than lung cancer revealed malignancies. None of the slides of nonsmokers who died of other causes showed signs of cancer.[93a]

It has been estimated that 98% of all lung cancer victims are smokers. Great Britain's Medical Research Council reported the risk of lung cancer above age 45 may be 50 times as great for those who smoke 25 cigarettes or more per day as for nonsmokers. The U.S. Surgeon General's Advisory Committee estimated the risk of dying of lung cancer is 18 times as great for heavy smokers as for nonsmokers in the 35 to 65 age group. For females the relationship is only slightly less pronounced. Fortunately though, when one quits smoking the risk declines to a level only slightly higher than that for those who never began smoking. Backing the epidemiological data are numerous studies with mice showing tobacco tars induce skin cancer. To date, however, researchers have not reported the appearance of lung cancer in laboratory animals into which cigarette smoke has been forced.[94]

A study of British vegans (strict vegetarians) indicates smoking is rare among these people. This was confirmed in private interviews. What's more surprising is that the near-vegetarian rural Abkhasians raise tobacco and yet few of them smoke. When smokers change to whole-food vegetarian diets, they usually lose the desire (need?) to smoke. Many Seventh Day Adventists are vegetarians and very few of this group smokes. It has been observed that smokers excrete significantly less vitamin C than nonsmokers, and smokers tend to take more sugar and coffee than nonsmokers. As with obesity, there may be too much emphasis on will power and not enough on the physiology of desire.[95]

While smoking seems to be the internal pollutant that ignites the overwhelming majority of the lung cancer fires, air pollution may also play a role. British Immigrants to South Africa have a much higher incidence of lung cancer than native-born white South Africans, and U.S. city-dwellers are reported to have a much higher incidence of lung cancer than do the handful still opting for country life. The highly carcinogenic polycyclic hydrocarbons are common air pollutants, and they have induced lung cancer in animals but they may be derived from foods, especially animal products, as well as polluted air.[96]

It is clear the most obvious way to avoid lung cancer is not to smoke. To this end a simple, vegetarian diet containing no stimulants or processed foods seems to offer promise. The death rate from lung cancer among Seventh Day Adventists is only 20% of that among non-Adventists.[97]

GASTROINTESTINAL SITES

About 100,000 new cases of cancer of the bowel (colon-rectum) and 30,000 new cases of stomach cancer are expected to be discovered in the U.S. during 1975. Bowel cancer is the most common form of cancer in the U.S.[98]

The incidence of bowel cancer among white Americans has changed little in recent years but the rate for blacks has grown steadily during the last decade. In 1937 the incidence for blacks was only about half the rate for whites, but by 1969 the rates were about the same. These trends are part of a tendency for blacks to "catch up" and be caught up in the mindless quest for more of everything with programmed preferences for hot dogs, apple pie and juicy steaks.[99]

It has already been pointed out that bile acids and other bile components including cholesterol may be transformed into powerful carcinogens in the intestines and that meat-eaters, possibly because of the high fat content of meat, pass abnormally large quantities of bile. The bile is secreted into the small intestines where, to be excreted in the feces, it must pass through the entire bowel (colon and rectum).[100]

Dr. Earnest L. Wynder, president of the American Health Foundation, links the high incidence of colon cancer in the U.S. to the surfeit of bile wastes resulting, he says, from the high fat intake of Americans. He acknowledges much of the fat is derived from the fat of beef and other meats, but he places no special significance in this. Others do.[101]

A study involving over 500 Japanese in Hawaii revealed a strong correlation between beef intake and bowel cancer but the correlation between total meat intake and the disease was even stronger.[102]

Dr. John W. Berg of the National Cancer Institute says "there is now substantial evidence that beef consumption is a key factor in determining bowel cancer incidence." Berg's contention is backed by (1) a strong correlation between beef consumption and bowel cancer among Japanese migrating to Hawaii during the 20's and 30's, (2) the observation that the Scots, who consume 19% more beef than the English, also have a 19% higher death rate from bowel cancer than do the English, (3) the high rates of bowel cancer in beef producing (and eating) nations and (4) the even higher rates of bowel cancer for heavy beef-eaters in beef producing nations.[103]

If fats and meat bring carcinogens into the bowel, the whole of the U.S. diet abets the work of these carcinogens. The lack of fiber (vitamin R) in sugar, refined grains, animal foods, vegetable protein extracts, etc., doubles the time it takes wastes to pass through the bowel, thus giving potential carcinogens twice the exposure time. A diet containing refined carbohydrates facilitated the appearance of colon tumors in rats, and rats were found to incur lower incidence of intestinal cancer on a high fibre diet even though their caloric intake was increased.[104]

It is not necessary to turn to the Hunzas or Abkhasians to find low incidences of bowel cancer. The disease is rare among Africans and Japanese in their native lands. When Africans and Japanese immigrate to the U.S. and adopt the diet of their host, however, the situation changes radically.[105]

Stomach cancer is declining in the United States but remains high in Iceland, Japan and Norway. Salted fish are common to the diets of all three nations and a high incidence of stomach cancer has been observed among those taking high quantities of salted, pickled vegetables and salted fish. Salted flesh foods are often smoked and hydrocarbons derived from smoking fish and meat have been implicated in stomach cancer also. It may be no coincidence that distaste for foods, especially meat, is an early symptom of stomach cancer. Heated fat and cholesterol have both produced stomach tumors in rats.[106]

In discussing the importance of the liver in preventing cancer, it was noted 100% of a group suffering from cancers of the gastrointestinal tract had liver disorders. Thus fats, meat, eggs, beef, sugar and other processed items, which have now been linked specifically to bowel and stomach cancer, may serve both to weaken the individual's resistance to gastrointestinal cancers and provide carcinogens to take advantage of that weakness.[107]

A DISTINCTLY MALE CANCER

The most common strictly male malignancy is cancer of the prostate gland: there were about 40,000 new cases discovered in 1969 and the incidence of prostate cancer is growing. It is estimated that a third to half of U.S. males reaching age 60 have enlarged prostates and though most enlarged prostates are not malignant, they can be forerunners of cancer and they are a source of much discomfort. Enlarged prostates have been related to stimulation by androgen (male sex) hormones even though androgen production is less in older men.[108]

Androgen hormones are produced from cholesterol and an excess of dietary cholesterol and saturated fat, both of which tend to elevate circulating cholesterol and might lead to an excessive production of androgen. The level of androgens might not be excessive were it possible for the elderly to engage in continued sex activity. But high-fat, high-protein diets, heavy laden with refined foods tend to lead to early "aging" (*see Chapter 4*) which fosters impotency.[109]

The early Incas were slow to develop as are now the rural Abkhasians. Relatively low in protein, fat and calories, their diets resulted in people capable of "physical marvels," but such diets do not lead to early physical maturity. Indeed, the male Abkhasians traditionally begin their sex life in their 30's but then continue until very advanced ages. The Incas reportedly married when men were in their mid 30's, women about 33. And there is every indication neither of these groups, or others eating simply, had any prostate problems.[110]

BLADDER CANCER

The urinary bladder was the site of an estimated 30,000 new cases of cancer in 1969. Three quarters of these occurred in males, and the incidence among males has been rising steadily in recent years. Bladder cancer is associated with urinary stones in rats and smokers have a significantly higher incidence of bladder cancer. Coffee drinking has also been implicated in bladder cancer.[111]

Urinary stones usually take the form of calcium and magnesium salts of phosphate or oxalate. For Americans, the deposits are likely to occur as acid ash calcium phosphate. Meat, eggs and dairy products are all high in phosphorus and all yield an acid ash. Calcium can reach the bladder from an excess of dietary calcium or from bone resorption brought on by high protein or high phosphorus intakes. Urinary stone patients have been treated with a diet low in dairy products and bladder tumors were elevated markedly in rats fed excess protein. Again, meat, eggs and dairy foods appear to be involved. Abandoning animal products and sugar may lower the risk further by eliminating the desire to smoke and drink coffee.[112]

ORAL CANCERS

There are about 27,000 cases of cancer of the mouth, pharynx and esophagus each year. Most cases are fatal and male victims outnumber female victims three to one. The incidence of these neoplasms is notably high among brewers, tavern keepers, bartenders and waiters, and cancers of the mouth and pharynx are said to occur almost exclusively in patients with histories of smoking and/or drinking but low molybdenum intake may be involved also. It is a bit inconsistent to disallow cigarette advertising while permitting a brewery to tell us it "still cares." But the brewers do not create the need for alcohol . . . we do, every time we eat a salted peanut, french fry or a hamburger. Without the salt there's no desire for any liquid: thirst is an unnecessary state, just as oral cancer is. A saltless whole-foods, vegetarian diet containing bean sprouts and greens prevents thirst, contains a rich supply of molybdenum and apparently ends the desire to smoke. Oral cancers are rare among the Seventh Day Adventists.[113]

TWO MORE ORGANS

Some 20,000 new cases of gallbladder and pancreatic cancer were recorded in 1969. As mentioned before gallbladder tumors are almost always preceded by gallstones. The latter, in turn, are usually preceded by liver disorders leading to excess bile output, decreased bile salt production, or both. It is well known that gallstones are "related to Western and European eating habits" and dieticians commonly recommend a low fat diet with limited intake of milk, eggs and butter for gallstones. Cholesterol and the bile acid, cholic acid, produced gallstones in mice and dogs while sugar and fat brought on gallstones in rabbits. Most cases of gallstones in the U.S. are cholesterol-based indicating animal products are involved. Animal products are further implicated by the fact that obesity raises the risk of gallstones.[114]

Cancer of the pancreas is often preceded by disturbed carbohydrate metabolism which can be avoided by low-fat, sugar-free diets. A significant relationship between meat intake and pancreatic cancer has been found in studies in Japan, and a low-calorie diet all but eliminated cancer of the pancreas in rats. It appears that steering away from animal products and processed items should protect against both gallbladder cancer and cancer of the pancreas.[115]

LEUKEMIA

The various forms of leukemia account for some 20,000 new cases

of cancer in the U.S. each year. Leukemia is associated with altera-
tions in the lymph glands, spleen, bone marrow and liver. The incidence of leukemia in rats can be cut substantially by restricting food
intake, and it was found that a low-fat diet delayed the appearance of
the disease in mice. A high incidence of leukemia was seen in animals
taking a diet containing 20% chicken fat. Low fat intake was very
effective in allowing mice to avoid tumors induced by ultraviolet
radiation, and leukemia has been linked to ultraviolet exposure as
well as viruses. It appears defense should be aimed at maintaining the
integrity of the liver and choosing a low-fat diet which prevents a
high caloric intake. The Seventh Day Adventists displayed a 38%
lower death rate from leukemia than non-Adventists.[116]

LIVER CANCER

Liver cancer, which has been linked to alcohol and other nutritional bombs, is declining in the U.S., but the disease continues to
plague groups like the Malasians and Bantu. When the Bantu start
eating "nutritionally adequate diets," however, their vulnerability to
liver tumors drops sharply. The change may be due to increased riboflavin in the liver. Good riboflavin sources (like sprouts and greens) .
tend to protect animals from cancer of the liver.[117]

Liver cancer is associated with processed food, excess calories and
excess protein in animals and high intake of alcohol in humans. We
may soon see a reversal of the decline in the incidence of liver cancer
in the U.S. unless the normal diet is altered markedly.[118]

CANCER TREATMENT

Today's cancer victim is faced with a strong possibility, if not cer-
tainty, of a most dreadful trek to early death. The surgeon's knife,
destruction of tissues by radiation and powerful drugs may add
months, or even years to the survival period for some, but those who
accede to such treatment are often left disfigured or incapacitated and
ripe for new neoplasms, or the reappearance of the ones so violently
exorcised.[119]

When, then, is it too late to reject the foods which produce "willing hosts" to cancer? A leading acupuncturist says cancer can be reversed when and if the liver can be regenerated. Gerson and Bieler
gave strong support to this contention and the vital role of the liver

in cancer has been firmly established by clinical findings. But if the liver is so vital in cancer why don't doctors treat the liver instead of, or in addition to, cutting or burning away tumors? There is interest along these lines and so-called bland diets may be the key to giving the liver the opportunity to repair itself so it can purge the body of cancer.[120]

Bieler treated a case of liver toxemia with an unsalted vegetable broth, a "desperately situated" case of liver malfunction with fruit juices and an inoperable cancer patient with an alkaline-ash vegan diet. All three recovered.[121]

T. L. O. Armstrong reported in New Zealand's *Soil and Health Journal* that a Hungarian doctor named Ferenczi reported good results from feeding ten lung cancer patients, four stomach cancer victims and other cancer patients with nothing but raw carrots for many months. The patients took about two pounds of carrots a day. Johanna Brandt brought world-wide attention to her "grape cure" for cancer; she recommends all kinds of grapes in unlimited quantities. Gerson used selected fruits and vegetables as the foundation for his treatment. He specifically chose fruits and vegetables low in sodium and having a high potassium-sodium ratio (e.g. eggplant, leeks, parsley, peas, potatoes, turnip greens, pumpkin, apples, grapes, plums, bananas, citrus fruit and melons) which he usually offered raw or in juice form. He sometimes added a little oatmeal to the diet, but no salt, sugar or milk, in or with, any food. Gerson used frequent enemas but warned against the administration of supplements.[122]

Growth promoting vitamins, minerals and protein supplements may accelerate the spread of cancer rather than slowing it. On the other hand, vitamin B_{17} (laetrile) is reported to have reversed many cases of human cancer. Grape seeds, which Johanna Brandt encouraged eating as part of the "grape cure," are a good source of laetrile and may be a big feature of her diet. The same may be true of selected foods employed by Gerson and others. Sprouts, especially mung bean sprouts like fruit seeds, are excellent sources of laetrile. Therefore, the SGA diet (possibly without seaweed) should be an exceptionally good diet for cancer patients.[123]

A competent acupuncturist may be able to gird the liver to repair itself and thus effect the disappearance of cancer. It stands to reason, however, that acupuncture could be even more effective if combined with the laetrile-rich SGA diet. In keeping with the patient's best interest any physician should advise those he treats to reform their eating habits, not for a prescribed period, but for the remainder of their lives.[124]

The cure rate with nonviolent methods should be taken in context: about 95% of Gerson's patients were "terminal" cases and Gerson testified before a Senate subcommittee in 1946 that he cured 30% of his "most hopeless cases." It certainly appears he did have a number of successes. In 1958, Gerson published a description of his treatment and a summary of 50 case histories. The subjects were, in all cases, patients who had been diagnosed and treated by one or more orthodox practitioners before coming to Gerson. Many had x-ray and/ or laboratory test results to verify they had cancer at the time they went to Gerson. Subsequent test results and testimony were offered to show the subjects responded to Gerson's diet and that almost all were free of cancer at the time his book was prepared.[125]

SUMMARY

Cancer is not inappropriately called "the disease of civilization." It seems to have been widespread in gluttonous Rome yet groups living and eating simply remain conspicuously free of cancer even today. At the cellular level cancer is seen as runaway growth: accelerated synthesis of ineffectual protein and rapid cell division. This suggests growth promoting diets, i.e. diets high in calories, animal protein and fat may be involved in the genesis of cancer.[126]

The Abkhasians and Hunzas remain free of cancer by taking essentially vegetarian diets based on unprocessed whole grains, vegetables, fruit and low-fat dairy products (in the case of the Abkhasians) and sprouts (in the case of the Hunzas). Their intakes of calories, fat, protein and cholesterol are much lower than those in America and they take no sugar and little or no salt. In nations where diets are low in animal products, fat, protein, calories and processed foods, cancer mortality rates are a fraction of those in Europe and the U.S. Vegetarians in the U.S. evidently enjoy a much lower death rate from cancer also.[127]

High caloric intake leads to a high incidence of all varieties of induced and spontaneous cancers in animals while low caloric intake results in sharp cuts in the incidence of animal cancers. Obesity is associated with a two- to-threefold increase in the incidence of cancer mortality among Westerners, and weight reductions to 20% below "normal" reduce the risk of cancer still further. High fat with at least modest levels of protein are strongly implicated in obesity, and fewer eating periods, unless extended to become periods of gorging, tend to lower caloric intake, hence tend to protect against obesity. Sugar, coffee and refined foods may also contribute to an excess of body fat.[128] 1881229

High fat intake, especially in the presence of a high level of protein, has been implicated directly in various cancers. Meat, eggs, whole milk, butter, cheese, etc., derive most of their calories from fat and contain substantial levels of protein which labels them prime suspects in cancer. Animal products are also high in potentially carcinogenic oleic acid and cholesterol. High temperatures may render animal products even greater threats: the drippings from barbecued meat can transform the meat into a most powerful cancer-causing vehicle. The high fat content of animal products tends to increase secretion of bile components which can be transformed into powerful carcinogens in the intestines.[129]

Evidently cancer can only occur when the integrity of the liver is impaired, and a liver secretion is believed to inhibit the development of tumors. High intake of fat-rich animal products, especially eggs, may cause liver degeneration and sugar is strongly implicated in liver impairment. Other refined foods also threaten the liver.[130]

Cooking any food destroys major portions of the water soluble vitamins necessary for proper liver function and overall body maintenance. Processing results in wholesale removal of vitamins and minerals from all foods. More than one group, including the Eskimos, remained free of cancer until they added sugar and refined flour to their diets.[131]

Assigning numerical ratios to the quality, degree of processing and amount of cooking seems to yield a good indication of the incidence of cancer among population groups. Highest ratings go to a strict vegetarian diet, high in sprouts and greens and eaten raw.[132]

The leading cancers have been related to specific factors: female cancers have been identified with excess food intake, high-fat, animal protein diets, formula feeding and promiscuity; sugar and salt may also be involved. Lung cancer is closely correlated with smoking, which in turn may result from stimulants such as coffee, sugar, medicines and alcohol and excesses, particularly meat. Bowel cancer has been tied to high fat intake, beef, sugar and refined foods; stomach cancer is much more prevalent when intake of smoked animal products and salted foods is high. Prostate cancer may be related to cholesterol intake and high-protein, high-fat diets, hence animal products. Urinary and gallbladder tumors have been associated with acid ash, animal products, coffee and smoking; oral cancers have been associated with alcohol and smoking. Pancreatic tumors have been linked to meat, and along with leukemia, have been linked to fat and sugar, while heptomas (liver cancers) are closely related to alcohol, fat, sugar, etc.[133]

The evidence that diet plays a key, if not dominant, role in all degenerative disease, including cancer, mounts daily. Total defense seems to be found in predominantly vegetarian diets containing no processed foods. Fat, sugar, eggs, meat, refined cereals, medicines, drugs and salt are probably the greatest contributors to cancer while a raw foods diet based on sprouted grains and beans, green vegetables and seaweed should lead to total protection. Though various vegetables, fruits, and juice diets seem to have cured many cancers, they are not always successful. The first order of business is prevention.[134]

There seems to be enough direct and epidemiological data linking cancer to the foundations of the American diet that researchers should be clamoring to set up studies in which groups volunteer to eat simple diets. The cost of such studies should be very low since simple foods are inherently inexpensive and volunteers should need no medical attention. The food of participants would require no elaborate preparation for cooking would be kept at a minimum. All that is required is scientists willing to search without prejudice about man's capacity for change.[134]

Hopefully, we will soon see "experimental" groups of volunteers undertake a diet of sprouts, greens and a little seaweed. The results of the trial are not likely to serve as a boon to the pocketbooks of meat packers, milk producers, brewers, millers, pharmacists, poultry farmers, politicians, physicians, restaurant owners, etc., but it should be a big boon to their health.[136]

2 / cardiovascular diseases

Cardiovascular diseases (diseases of the heart and blood vessels) are responsible for half the deaths in America. The leading cardiovascular killer is coronary heart disease: the average man of age 40 is reported to have about a one-in-three chance of having a "coronary" before age 50. Coronary heart disease has been called "the most important health problem in developed societies" but cerebral vascular seizures, or strokes, take a heavy toll also. The five leading cardiovascular disorders, which account for over 90% of deaths attributed to the heart and blood vessels, are listed below.[137]

Disease	Estimated annual death toll in the United States
Coronary Heart disease (Heart attacks)	560,000
Cerebral vascular disease (Strokes)	200,000
Hypertension (High blood pressure)	70,000
Myocardial (Heart muscle) degeneration	50,000
Arteriosclerosis (Hardening of the arteries)	40,000

The origin of coronary heart disease, cerebral vascular disease, arteriosclerosis, and to some extent, every other form of cardiovascular disease is a condition called atherosclerosis. Atherosclerosis begins as a build-up of fatty deposits along the artery walls. The fatty deposits are believed to arise from cholesterol and other fat-related substances in the blood but in time the deposits accumulate calcium and other minerals. The deposits reach the stage of atherosclerosis when the mineral content is sufficient to cause hardening. The hardened fatty deposits, that is atherosclerosis, tend to become more pronounced and widespread with age and the main artery of the body, the aorta, is often affected.[138]

When atherosclerosis becomes very pronounced, blood passing through the affected arteries is likely to form clots, a condition known as thrombosis. When clotting and blockage occurs in vessels leading to the heart the condition is called "coronary thrombosis," which is the most common form of fatal heart attacks. When clotting and blockage takes place in arteries leading to a portion of the brain the condition is called "cerebral thrombosis," which is what most strokes are.[139]

Clots do not always shut off blood flow completely, and sometimes a piece of a clot will break off and be carried along until it reaches and plugs a smaller artery. This form of blockage constitutes another way in which coronaries or strokes can occur. Pieces of clots can also lodge in arteries leading to the kidneys, spleen, lungs or liver. When this happens, the affected organ, or the portion of that organ dependent on blood from the affected artery, ceases to function.[140]

Atherosclerosis weakens the walls of arteries and affected arteries may rupture and bleed (hemorrhage). Strokes often take the form of cerebral hemorrhages resulting from rupture of arteries which supply blood to the brain.[141]

There is very strong evidence that atherosclerosis is derived from fat-related substances (lipids) in the blood. The serum concentrations of the principle lipid constituents of atherosclerotic deposits, cholesterol, which occurs only in animals, and triglycerides, which are the essence of all dietary fats and oils, are closely correlated to the degree of atherosclerosis in humans. Moreover, the lipid composition of atherosclerotic deposits tends to match the lipid composition of the blood. The links between serum cholesterol and atherosclerosis can hardly be casual: high serum cholesterol is followed by atherosclerosis in rabbits, dogs, monkeys and other animals and the transfer of serum cholesterol to atherosclerotic build-ups has been traced by the use of radioactive substances in humans.[142]

At the present time there is no accurate and dependable way to observe atherosclerotic build-ups in the arteries of live human beings. However, serum cholesterol and serum triglyceride levels offer reasonably reliable indications of the overall degree of atherosclerosis present. The serum levels of the two lipids allow physicians to gauge the risk of impending heart attacks and other cardiovascular seizures, but the risk is markedly increased by other factors including obesity, impaired carbohydrate metabolism, high blood pressure and smoking.[143]

Autopsies on the bodies of 300 U.S. soldiers killed in the Korean War showed 77% had severe atherosclerosis and the condition is developing in ever younger Americans and Europeans each decade. Some ten years after the Korean war study, autopsies were performed on the bodies of 350 Bostonians, and it was discovered all who were beyond the age of thirty had developed a degree of atherosclerosis. A recent study indicates damage to the coronary arteries may now be starting to appear in young children in Europe. A noted authority on heart disease said atherosclerosis "is simply one of the accompaniments of adult life," but the statement is valid only insofar as it applies to inhabitants of the industrialized nations consuming a large quantity of animal products.[144]

In their popular and very useful book on heart care, Drs. Blakeslee and Stamler noted that there is rarely a significant degree of atherosclerosis in individuals taking vegetarian diets low in calories, total fat, saturated fat and cholesterol. (It should be pointed out, though, that such diets are often low in refined foods, especially sugar.) The African Bantu, who take very small quantities of meat, dairy products and refined foods, remain "remarkably free from atherosclerosis" while at least one African tribe which takes a great deal of animal food is reported to have high levels of serum cholesterol and a high incidence of coronary heart disease. Israeli Temenites, who take only about half as much animal protein as European-born Israelis, incur a far less degree of atherosclerosis than their European-born fellow countrymen. California Seventh Day Adventists have mortality rates from coronary heart disease and strokes roughly half that of comparable non-Adventists. These findings are remarkable since only about half of the Adventists are believed to be vegetarian. The life expectancy of Adventists is also considerably longer than that of non-Adventists.[145]

The Abkhasians take no sugar or refined grains and take flesh products only once or twice a week, and a nine-year study of Centenarians in Abkhasia indicates atherosclerosis is rare in those people. The Vilcabambas are said to take less animal food than the Abkhasians and a report from an American physician who observed both groups suggests the Vilcabambas are, like the Abkhasians, highly resistant to cardiovascular disease. As a rule the Hunzas take meat only once a year, and a renowned British physician who spent ten years with the Hunzas, reported he never witnessed a heart attack or a stroke during his visit.[146]

The Japanese take far less animal food and sugar than Americans and though most Japanese seem to eventually develop atherosclerosis, its progression was found tó lag that of Americans by 20 years or more on the average. The previously mentioned autopsies on the bodies of 350 Bostonians were part of a comparative study which included examinations of the arteries of 352 deceased Japanese in Fukuka. The study showed the average American of age 40 had a degree of atherosclerosis comparable to that of the average Japanese at age 60. Some rather elderly Japanese were entirely free of atherosclerosis while none of the Americans past the age of 30 were free of the condition.[147]

While no group taking primarily vegetarian unprocessed foods has ever been found to have a high incidence of coronary heart disease, at least two groups who take a large amount of raw flesh and blood were reported to avoid heart seizures. The African Masai, who drink the fresh blood and milk of their herds are said to retain low levels of serum cholesterol and avoid coronaries while the Eskimos, who took a large amount of raw fish and blubber, seem to have been free from symptoms of cardiovascular disease in general. However, these findings should not be taken to mean high levels of flesh and blood, even when taken raw, are desirable. Until early adulthood Masai males take a mixed diet, and it is only during a two-year stint as warriors that they attempt to live on animal products alone. Following their warrior period the Masai decline dramatically and though still in their 20's they look and act old, and rely on their women, who raise and eat plant foods, to sustain them. The Eskimos also decline in their 20's and have a life expectancy of under 30 years. The climate of the Eskimos can hardly explain their shortened life expectancy for the long living (almost totally vegetarian) Hunzas endure a climate only slightly less severe. There is something to be learned from the Eskimos and Masai but it is not how to avoid degeneration.[148]

SERUM CHOLESTEROL

The American Medical Association (AMA) in conjunction with the National Academy of Sciences, placed elevated blood lipids, especially cholesterol, at the top of its list of "risk factors" in coronary heart disease. The AMA noted only a third of U.S. men have a serum cholesterol level under 220 milligrams percent (that is 220 milligrams per 100 milliliters). Groups taking little animal food and having low incidences of cardiovascular disease tend to maintain serum cholesterol levels 180 milligrams percent. The Bantu are reported to have serum cholesterol levels as low as 95 milligrams percent. Evidently these low serum cholesterol findings are simply reflections of dietary differences for when groups of Bantu and White South African volunteers were given the same diets there were no differences in serum lipid patterns of the two groups.[149]

Long term studies indicate keeping serum cholesterol under 220, as suggested by the AMA, might cut the incidence of heart attacks in half while bringing the level under 200 should reduce the incidence fourfold; lowering levels to the 150 to 180 range without the use of drugs might bring an end to America's biggest killer. Instead of decreasing their serum cholesterol though, most North Americans are letting their levels grow with age. The average for North American men is probably about 200 milligrams percent at age 20, over 220 by age 30, and 240 or more in middle age. The increase parallels the build-up of atherosclerosis and is not seen in groups who avoid atherosclerosis.[150]

The AMA suggests that to reduce serum cholesterol, individuals should reduce their intake of cholesterol and fats, especially saturated fats. Most of the saturated fat and all of the cholesterol in the American diet is derived from animal products: eggs, meat, milk, cheese, fish, etc. It is thus not surprising that controlled experiments have shown eliminating animal products from diets tends to bring about very favorable reductions in serum cholesterol.[151]

After only two weeks on strict vegetarian diets the serum cholesterol of a group of young women fell from 182 milligrams percent to 140 milligrams percent, and the levels of middle-aged men fell from 295 milligrams percent to 172 milligrams percent. The levels of both groups remained low until they returned to their former diets. Similar results were found with a group of men 23 to 30 years of age and after a three-and-a-half year search for a diet to keep serum lipids down, Dr. Endel Kask of the Metropolitan State Hospital in Norwalk, California arrived at a "very strict vegetarian diet." Vegans are reported to have markedly lower serum cholesterol levels than individuals who include animal products in their diets. British physicians found a group of vegans had an average serum cholesterol level of 181 milligrams percent whereas a comparable group of individuals taking normal diets had a level of 240 milligrams percent.[152]

It appears that any reduction in consumption of animal products, especially meat and eggs, tends to have a favorable affect on serum cholesterol. A group of Norwegian males of middle age or beyond who followed lacto-vegetarian diets, that is, a vegetarian diet in which one abstains from meat, eggs and fish but partakes of dairy products, had serum cholesterol levels of 198 milligrams percent compared to 260 milligrams percent for Norwegian meat-eating men of the same ages. A study involving 233 U.S. vegetarians and 283 meat-eaters showed that serum cholesterol levels increased as the degree of nonvegetarianism increased. This has been verified in studies in which the serum cholesterol levels of vegans, lacto-vegetarians and meat-eaters are compared. The results of a study by two Harvard professors are given below:[153]

	Serum Cholesterol Levels (mg per 100 ml)		
	Vegans	Lacto-Vegetarians	Meat-Eaters
Men	206	243	288
Women	206	269	295

A team of researchers at Peter Bent Brigham Hospital in Boston showed how quickly meat can affect serum cholesterol by putting 12 volunteers with comparatively low (215 milligrams percent) serum cholesterol levels on the meat-rich Stillman diet. After an average of only 7.6 days serum cholesterol levels of the volunteers had jumped to 248 milligrams percent. Clearly the price of meat and milk is more than the currency turned over to the grocer.[154]

Most researchers believe high serum cholesterol results primarily from dietary cholesterol and fats, especially fats rich in saturated fatty acids such as lard, tallow, butter and grease. Fatty acids are called saturated when they are unable to take on additional hydrogen ions; fats rich in the saturated fatty acids tend to be solid at room temperature and are called saturated fats. Common vegetable oils such as corn oil, safflower oil, sunflower oil, sesame oil, soybean oil and olive oil are rich in highly unsaturated (polyunsaturated) fatty acids and are thus called polyunsaturated fats. Polyunsaturated fats tend to lower serum cholesterol when substituted for saturated fats in the diet, but high intake of fats *per se* tends to elevate serum cholesterol and increase the risk of atherosclerosis.[155]

Most saturated fats are derived from meat and dairy products; common meats and cheeses derive 40% to 80% of their total calories from saturated fats while milk and eggs derive about 50% of their total calories from saturated fats. Fowl contain lesser amounts of saturated fats and white fish are fairly low in saturated fats. Butter and tallow are almost pure saturated fats. Vegetables, grains, legumes and fruit normally derive less than 10% calories from fat and less than 3% of their calories from saturated fats. Oilseeds and nuts derive up to 90% of their calories from fat but saturated fats seldom exceed 20% of the calories in these foods.[156]

No plant food contains any cholesterol while all animal products contain cholesterol. Eggs, liver and certain sea foods contain the greatest quantities but all meats, dairy products, fish, fowl, animal fats and low-fat animal products contain sizeable quantities of cholesterol.[157]

ELEVATED SERUM CHOLESTEROL

Defenders of the American way of eating are quick to point out that cholesterol has a useful purpose in the body: it is a constituent of the protective coating surrounding nerve fibers and serves as the building block for various substances, including sex hormones. The normal liver synthesizes cholesterol and empties it into the blood stream so the appearance of cholesterol in the blood is a natural phenomena. But a high level of serum cholesterol is not a natural phenomenon. And every milligram of dietary cholesterol tends to boost blood levels, increase body accumulations and raise the risk of atherosclerosis.[158]

To gauge the effect of dietary cholesterol on serum cholesterol in humans, a number of men were put on cholesterol-free diets for 21 days, then divided into four groups with various fixed cholesterol intakes for 42 days. The resulting serum cholesterol levels are given below:[159]

Serum Cholesterol Levels
v.s. Dietary Cholesterol Levels

Number of Men	Cholesterol Intake (mg/1000 cal)	Serum Cholesterol Levels (mg percent)	Changes from 21st day (mg/100 ml)
18	0	164.7	+ 3.4
11	106	174.7	+13.0
13	212	181.1	+23.8
14	317	198.4	+40.5

A group of researchers at Harvard verified these findings and reported the effect of dietary cholesterol is independent of the effect of saturated fat in diet. This implies that cholesterol in its natural state, that is with saturated fats, is worse than cholesterol alone. The average cholesterol intake in America is sufficient to guarantee a high level of serum cholesterol, and differences in serum cholesterol levels between a cholesterol-free diet and normal diets could represent the differences between freedom from coronary heart disease and high risk of heart attacks.[160]

Eggs are the richest source of cholesterol in the diets of most Americans, and eggs may play an important role in high serum cholesterol and atherosclerosis. A diet of mainly boiled eggs induced "accelerated atherosclerosis lesions" in cockerels. The serum cholesterol levels of the egg-eating cockerels were five to ten times those of controls. Rhesus monkeys had enormous increases in serum cholesterol and severe atherosclerosis in the aorta after 12 weeks on egg yolk powder and butter as 40% of their calories. Adding eggs to diets of individuals who are already taking high levels of saturated fats and cholesterol seems to boost the serum cholesterol of only a portion of those involved, but the addition of eggs, or food containing eggs, to diets rich in vegetable oils nullified the serum cholesterol lowering effects of the polyunsaturated fats.[161]

It certainly appears diets aimed at checking the degree of atherosclerosis should call for sharply reducing, if not eliminating, dietary cholesterol. The first step in that direction is to eliminate eggs from the diet. It is heartening to note that monkeys lost much of the cholesterol in atherosclerotic plaques built by a diet high in cholesterol when cholesterol was eliminated from their diet.[162]

Saturated fats are at least as potent as cholesterol in elevating serum cholesterol and causing atherosclerosis. Diets containing relatively modest levels of saturated fat cause remarkable rises in the serum cholesterol of animals, and lard is used as a standard vehicle for inducing experimental atherosclerosis in rats. Predictably saturated fats cause heart seizures in animals also.[163]

Experiments with groups of young men showed substituting corn oil for saturated fat as 40% of calories resulted in substantial reductions in serum cholesterol. Substituting cottonseed oil for whole milk, cream or butter led to significantly lower serum cholesterol in volunteers at Tulane University and replacing meat and dairy products with fish and corn oil lowered the serum cholesterol of volunteers in Romania.[164]

Such findings should not be interpreted as meaning a high level of any kind of fat is not harmful. High levels of vegetable oil have resulted in heart lesions and elevated serum cholesterol in rats and peanut oil has led to atherosclerosis in monkeys and rats. Atherosclerosis patients and normal adults both experienced reductions in serum cholesterol when their total fat intake was reduced. Reductions matched those obtained from substituting polyunsaturated fats for saturated fats. In a long term study involving young males with coronary heart disease, it was found that lowering total fat intake from 45% to 28% of calories brought about marked reductions in recurrent heart attacks and mortality rates. Merely substituting polyunsaturated fats for saturated fats in their diets did not influence serum cholesterol or mortality. Generally though, the substitution of polyunsaturated fats for saturated fats does reduce serum cholesterol, and when the substitution is combined with cuts in total fat and cholesterol, serum cholesterol levels tend to fall precipitously and remain low as long as the changes are continued.[165]

A renowned Finnish researcher, Dr. M. J. Karvonen, reported in the proceedings of the Nutrition Society that decreasing the saturated fat content of the diet is twice as effective in lowering serum cholesterol as increasing the amount of polyunsaturated fats. He emphasized the need for cutting the level of saturated fats, which for Westerners means cutting total fat intake, rather than just adding polyunsaturates. Two pathologists from Cambridge University have recommended that, "Saturated fats and cholesterol containing foods, for instance, cream, eggs and butter, should be completely omitted from the diet." In essence, they are suggesting a switch to a strict vegetarian diet.[166]

While most animal products are high in saturated fats and cholesterol which promote high serum cholesterol and atherosclerosis, many unprocessed plant foods contain substances which act to keep serum cholesterol down. One important cholesterol lowering factor is crude fiber or vitamin R (from "Roughage"). Lack of vitamin R leads to an intestinal disorder known as diverticular disease, and the growth of diverticular disease has paralleled the rise in coronary heart disease in the West. The rural Bantu, who have remarkably low serum cholesterol and a very low incidence of cardiovascular disease, take about 25 grams of vitamin R per day which is at least four times the amount available in normal U.S. foods. Processing removes most of the vitamin R from grains while animal products, oils, sugar and salt contain no crude fiber so the diets of many Americans may be almost void of the vitamin. On the other hand, American vegetarians tend to avoid processed foods and (vitamin R-free) animal products so that their vitamin R intake is on a par with that of the rural Bantu.[167]

Experiments in Holland and India showed serum cholesterol levels were lowered substantially when a sizeable amount of vitamin R-rich rolled oats replaced an equivalent amount of white bread or when a large quantity of beans was included in the diets of volunteers. A British study was less conclusive but all parties involved may have been taking adequate amounts of vitamin R.[168]

The serum cholesterol lowering effects of whole rice, corn, barley, wheat, and oats as opposed to refined forms of the same grains has been demonstrated in animals fed pure cholesterol or eggs. Vitamin R-rich alfalfa, wheat straw, peat and leguminous seeds all afforded rabbits considerable protection against atherosclerosis. Supplements of vitamin R-rich rice bran effected a marked reduction in the serum cholesterol of cholesterol-fed rats but the drop was far less than with whole rice.[169]

The process by which whole-plant foods or the vitamin R of such foods lowers serum cholesterol is not clear. However, the liver breaks down cholesterol to produce bile acids which are excreted into the intestine, and there is evidence an increase of fiber in the intestine leads to increased production of bile acids, hence increased removal of cholesterol from the blood by the liver. In any event, whole-plant foods rich in vitamin R do tend to lower serum cholesterol.[170]

While the starch of refined grains tends to elevate serum cholesterol, another carbohydrate, sucrose (sugar), has an adverse effect on serum cholesterol levels. The serum cholesterol level of sugar-fed animals tends to be higher than for animals fed (cholesterol raising) refined starches. The differences can be reduced, but not eliminated by supplemental chromium. Not surprisingly rabbits fed diets high in both sugar and saturated fat (such as beef tallow) developed severe atherosclerosis; they had their life spans cut in half. Russian researchers have discovered that a low-cholesterol, low-fat diet is ineffective for heart patients when it includes six ounces of sugar daily (average intake in North America is five ounces per day). When starch replaces sugar in their diet, however, serum lipids fall and the threat of clotting is reduced.[171]

Often appearing in the diet with sugar is caffeine which may also be a contributor to the problem of high serum cholesterol. Heart attack victims were found to drink more coffee than others, and the addition of coffee to the diet of rats elevated serum cholesterol. There is evidence the rise resulted from the caffeine in coffee. Thus, cola drinks are implicated on two counts: sugar and caffeine.[172]

A digestible (and reportedly delectable) carbohydrate called guar gum has also been found to be very effective in lowering serum cholesterol. Guar gum is found in seaweeds and rats fed seaweeds had substantial reductions in serum cholesterol. Soviet researchers added a salad containing seaweed to the diets of 50 atherosclerosis patients and found a marked improvement in the ability of the small arteries to supply blood to the body.[173]

Cholesterol-lowering seaweed is an integral part of the SGA diet, and the SGA diet offers an abundant amount of vitamin R. The SGA diet contains no sugar, caffeine or cholesterol, and it is extremely low in saturated fats. Calorie for calorie the SGA diet contains at least three times as much manganese, magnesium, chromium, potassium, folacin, pantothenic acid, pyridoxine, niacin and riboflavin as the normal U.S. diet. All of these nutrients may aid in keeping serum cholesterol down and preventing atherosclerosis.[174]

Dietary manganese reportedly lowers the serum cholesterol and reduces the degree of atherosclerosis in rabbits. Magnesium deficiency enhanced sclerotic build-ups in the hearts of mice, and it has been suggested human atherosclerosis may be tied to chromium deficiency. Chronic potassium deficiency is alleged to play a role in degeneration of the heart and blood vessels also. A low level potassium diet is exacerbated by the use of (totally unnecessary) salt. Sodium from table salt increases the excretion of potassium and tends to replace potassium in the cells.[175]

Supplemental folacin improved the blood flow of elderly atherosclerosis patients, and a diet containing 5% dried mushrooms, which are rich in pantothenic acid dramatically lowered the serum cholesterol of rats. Pyridoxine-deficient monkeys develop atherosclerosis rapidly and niacin, riboflavin and vitamin C have all been used to lower serum cholesterol levels of humans. Atherosclerosis reportedly accumulates in tissues where a great deal of vitamin A is stored, and quail chicks developed increased build-ups of atherosclerosis when their vitamin A intake was lowered.[176]

With every new finding concerning the capacity of specific nutrients to lower serum cholesterol and reduce atherosclerosis the advantages of a vegan diet of the SGA type mount. But the absence of cholesterol, sugar and refined foods and remarkably low levels of saturated fats and total fats in such diets seem to be the real keys to their protective capacities.[177]

ELEVATED SERUM TRIGLYCERIDES

So far the discussion of cardiovascular disease has centered on serum cholesterol levels as an indication of the degree of atherosclerosis present. It may be recalled, however, that atherosclerotic deposits contain triglycerides as well as cholesterol, and the level of serum triglycerides is another important indicator of the extent of the build-ups. Sometimes patients with severe atherosclerosis have relatively low serum cholesterol levels but such patients invariably exhibit elevated serum triglycerides. Thus atherosclerosis may be regarded advanced when either serum cholesterol or serum triglycerides are high.[178]

Studies indicate the serum triglyceride levels of individuals susceptible to coronaries are seldom less than 160 milligrams percent and usually exceed 180 milligrams percent. Sobering it is then to find the average level of a large group of presumably normal Canadian civil servants in their late 30's exceeded 200 milligrams percent. The levels of 22-year-old Canadian civil servants averaged 120 milligrams percent, suggesting that in North America serum triglyceride concentrations rise even more markedly than serum cholesterol with age. There is no evidence of such rises in individuals on whole foods, more vegetarian diets, however. And switches to sugar-free vegetarian diets have resulted in dramatic drops in serum triglycerides.[179]

A sugar-free vegan diet containing soybean products, cereals, breads, vegetables and fruits resulted in a drop in serum triglyceride levels from 160 milligrams percent to only 76 milligrams percent for six male volunteers at a prison in Iowa. The serum triglycerides of the prisoners remained extraordinarily low even when a large amount of fat was added to their diet. When sugar replaced starch in their diet, however, serum triglyceride levels soared to 208 milligrams percent. Researchers in North Carolina found various vegan diets containing large amounts of wheat starch resulted in lower serum triglycerides for young adults, and a group of 31 healthy lacto-vegetarian males in Norway had serum triglyceride readings of only 65 milligrams percent. The lacto-vegetarians were taking considerably more dietary starch than ordinary Norwegians and their sugar intake was relatively low. These findings suggest sugar may be the principle cause of elevated serum triglycerides and this is supported by numerous research findings with animals and humans.[180]

When sugar was substituted for starch in the diet of rats, the quantity of triglycerides emptied into the blood doubled and studies show various animals including monkeys experience significant increases in serum triglycerides when sugar is substituted for starch in their diets. Supplemental chromium has failed to offset the effect of high sugar intake.[181]

Human studies include one in which 13 men experienced a drop in serum triglycerides from 232 milligrams percent to 162 milligrams percent when they cut their sugar intake in half. In other studies it was found replacing sugar with starch in the diets of normal British and American volunteers, subjects with high serum lipids in San Francisco and Israel and Venezuelan patients with coronary heart disease, all brought about substantial reductions in serum triglycerides. In other experiments it was found substituting sugar for starch, sugar for starch and fat or sugar for fat alone, resulted in elevated serum triglycerides in men. In still another experiment, sugar seemed to have a greater effect on the serum triglycerides of patients already suffering from abnormally high serum triglycerides than those of normal individuals.[182]

Authorities generally agree that "carbohydrate inducible" varieties of high serum triglycerides are common, especially among individuals with clinical atherosclerosis.[183]

At least one experiment showed serum triglyceride levels were unaffected by a shift from sugar to starch. However, the starch was derived from refined foods and it has been shown purified starch can cause even greater increases in the serum triglycerides of rabbits than sugar. It is reported older persons taking high levels of refined carbohydrates of any kind tend to have an exceptionally high number of cardiovascular disorders.[184]

The effect of fat and dietary cholesterol on serum triglyceride levels is not entirely clear. However, experiments do indicate individuals are more susceptible to effects of sugar when taking high levels of saturated fat and cholesterol or simply high levels of fat. Marked thinness is said to be uniformly associated with lower serum triglycerides, and low-fat diets tend to promote loss of weight which tends to bring about sustained reductions in serum triglyceride levels. On the other hand a recent study showed weight losses attained through high meat intake were accompanied by no reductions in serum triglycerides. Vegetable oils show some tendency to result in lower serum triglycerides than animal fats, but the results are not uniform.[185]

The problem of elevated serum triglycerides is clearly and strongly related to high intake of sugar and other refined carbohydrates. High fat intake, especially saturated fats, may also contribute to the problem. This implies diets designed to prevent cardiovascular disease should be free of refined foods, especially sugar.[186]

Studies at the Institute of Nutrition and Medical Science in Moscow, the University of Colorado and at two Helsinki mental hospitals showed lowering fat and cholesterol intake is far more effective in treating and preventing coronary heart disease when sugar intake is also reduced.[187]

There is some evidence refined carbohydrates, especially sugar, can cause human atherosclerosis even when the diet is relatively low in animal products but high intakes of both animal products and refined carbohydrates must be regarded as a far greater danger.[188]

That atherosclerosis is related to serum levels of cholesterol and triglycerides which depend on diet is beyond question. This does not imply however, the fat and cholesterol we eat simply floats in the blood until it finds a convenient spot to attack the arteries. Such a simplistic view is obviously false from the observations that sugar (a carbohydrate) leads to elevated serum triglycerides (fats) and saturated fats lead to elevated serum cholesterol (a fat-related substance, but not a fat).[189]

Dietary cholesterol does tend to boost serum cholesterol, of course, but this is simply because the liver does not slow down its net output of cholesterol enough to accommodate the dietary load. In addition to producing the cholesterol that elevates serum cholesterol, the liver also converts sugar into triglycerides which leads to the rise in serum triglycerides following a sugar load. This does not mean atherosclerosis begins as a liver disease: the human liver was simply not designed for the extremes to which normal Western diets subject it. Indeed, high intakes of eggs, sugar or alcohol have been shown to lead to fatty livers in rats. Naturally, the damaged liver is apt to be less capable of dealing with subsequent dietary overloads so either the liver or the cardiovascular system, or both, may be subjected to accelerated degeneration. Liver damage is associated with all manner of degenerative disease including cancer and diabetes. The key to a strong liver is abstinence from drugs and a diet which is rich in all the necessary vitamins, minerals and amino acids, but which contains no sugar or refined carbohydrates (including alcohol) and little animal fat, total fat or cholesterol.[190]

Only with a whole-foods vegan diet is one completely freed of the effects of refined foods and foods of animal origin. And only with carefully chosen vegan diets is one guaranteed a low total fat intake and a full supply of necessary nutrients and factors which actively abate atherosclerosis. Thus what's good for the arteries is good for the liver and conversely.[191]

HYPERTENSION

Hypertension (high blood pressure) alone takes considerably more lives than automobile accidents, and it greatly increases the risk of other cardiovascular diseases and dims the chances of recovery for those who survive a seizure. After following the incidence of coronary heart disease among Framingham, Massachusetts adults for eight years, it was concluded the risk of developing coronary heart disease with a systolic blood pressure (pressure of the blood leaving the heart) of 180 millimeter Hg or more was eight times as high as with a systolic pressure less than 120 millimeter Hg. British researchers found that patients who recover from their first stroke can usually avoid a second seizure if their blood pressure is brought down substantially. When their blood pressure remains high, however, fewer than one-in-five can expect to escape a second stroke or a heart attack.[192]

Like other factors associated with cardiovascular diseases, the blood pressure of North Americans and Europeans worsens with age. The systolic pressure of young adults normally lies in the range of 100 to 120 millimeters Hg, but for most it rises to 140 or more by the time they reach their 50's. Some researchers regard anything above 130 as high. Others use a different criteria but as one authority puts it, "the lower the pressure, the better."[193]

In some individuals there is no rise in blood pressure with age and low blood pressure in middle age is the rule in many parts of Africa and Asia. The blood pressure of Abkhasians in their 80's and beyond remains low while the blood pressure of the natives of New Guinea actually falls with advancing age.[194]

Northern Japanese farmers are said to have the highest blood pressure in the world and their salt intake, which averages about five teaspoons per day, is believed to be the highest in the world. Hypertension is less extreme, but still widespread, in Southern Japan where salt intake is a high two-to-three teaspoons per day. Nearby, in China, inlanders traditionally use no salt and blood pressures evidently remain low. Salt intake also tends to be low in regions of Africa and Asia where blood pressure usually remains low. High salt intake appears to be accompanied by high blood pressure in other regions of Africa. The Abkhasians take very little salt and rarely develop high blood pressure while New Guineans who enjoy a decline in blood pressure with age, use no salt at all and take a diet which provides as little as 70 milligrams of sodium per day. That is less than two percent of the average U.S. intake and one percent of what the U.S. army seems to believe necessary, but there is no evidence of sodium deficiency among the New Guineans.[195]

When the cells of the muscle of the artery walls accumulate sodium, the muscles contract and constrict the arteries, thus forcing a rise in blood pressure. Removal of the sodium from the artery wall cells requires a pumping action that depends on stimulation by a hormone produced by the kidneys, and therefore, kidney insufficiency can lead to accumulation of sodium in the artery walls which results in hypertension. Kidney insufficiency may in turn result from an inadequate supply of blood to the kidneys as a result of atherosclerosis.[196]

Since high blood pressure is quite common and clear-cut cases of kidney insufficiency are uncommon, many cases of high blood pressure occur in the presence of normal kidney activity. Nevertheless salt may still be involved, for high salt-intake leads to increased water retention, hence a dilution of nutrient concentrations in the blood. It is hypothesized that demand for increased blood-flow to maintain the supply of nutrients at needed levels leads to constriction of peripheral arteries which in turn elevates blood pressure.[197]

Regardless of the mechanism by which salt tends to elevate blood pressure, there is a much higher sodium content in the arteries of patients and animals with hypertension and these levels return to normal when the hypertension is relieved. Various animals experience substantial increases in blood pressure on diets with added salt. Typical Japanese diets lead to high blood pressure in at least one strain of rats and very high levels of salt tend to promote rapid increases in blood pressure, kidney damage and injury to other organs of various animals. A Soviet researcher reported salt concentrations in excess of 2.5 grams per liter (roughly the amount in the U.S. diet) produced "distinct hypertensive effect" in experimental animals.[198]

Dr. Lewis K. Dahl and a colleague at the Brookhaven National Laboratories found the incidence of high blood pressure among laboratory employees who habitually added salt to their food was 15 times as great as the incidence among employees who never added salt to their food. A Russian physician, Dr. V. A. Zusmanovich confirmed the relationship between hypertension and the habit of adding salt to food for individuals involved in mental activity, but not for individuals doing physical work. "Low-sodium" diets have led to improved kidney function and strengthened metabolic performance for patients with hypertension, and when patients with various cardiovascular disorders were given sodium-restricted diets as part of their treatment they experienced not only improved circulation but lower blood pressure as well.[199]

Salt has been linked to more than just hypertension: salt is believed to elevate serum triglycerides and be a possible factor in coronary heart disease in humans.[200]

The SGA diet contains no salt but it contains abundant amounts of the minerals present in salt, namely sodium and chlorine. Dietary salt is at best unnecessary and, it is clear it can be very harmful. Americans take an estimated 14 grams of salt per day which gives them a sodium intake up to 50 times their needs. Without salt, however, the U.S. diet might be deficient in iodine, which is added to salt. The SGA diet derives a great surplus of iodine from the tiny amount of seaweed it includes.[201]

Sprouts, raw vegetables and fresh fruits are very high in water so when taken without salt, there is neither desire nor need for liquid. Individuals taking the SGA diet experience no thirst even after strenuous exercise in hot climates. Dependence on water can lead to hypertension via increased water retention.[202]

Those who continue to eat foods which require salt for palatability might be wise to at least avoid chlorinated tap water. An independent physician, Dr. J. M. Price, reported high concentrations of chlorine in water led to severe atherosclerosis in cockerels. Rats evidently do not react to chlorine in the same way, but the issue is disturbingly unclear for humans. The rise in coronary heart disease in North America and Europe has paralleled the spread of chlorination.[203]

Salt is not the only cause of hypertension. Anything which interferes with arterial blood flow or kidney function can induce hypertension. The arterial pressure of rabbits was elevated by high fat intake, and researchers suspect magnesium deficiency may lead to reduced activity of the pump that removes sodium from artery walls. The affects of high salt intake may be aggravated by low calcium intake, and an inadequate intake of niacin may facilitate an increase in blood pressure for individuals under stress.[204]

High protein intake has caused increased blood pressure in normal rats and humans with liver diseases. High protein intake adversely affected the kidneys of obese women and low-protein diets are being employed on an increasing scale to treat kidney insufficiency. A potato diet has been quite effective in taking the strain off of damaged kidneys.[205]

Animal products would appear to have no place in a diet designed to treat high blood pressure. They are inherently high in sodium and contain high quantities of fat and/or protein. Animal products are poor sources of magnesium and except for dairy products, they tend to be poor sources of calcium. It is not surprising then, that salt-free vegan diets have been employed in treating high blood pressure.[206]

A group of South African researchers headed by Dr. B. J. Meyer found a fruit and nut diet was effective in reducing the blood pressure of humans, and Kempner employed his diet of unsalted white rice, fruit and sugar with vitamins and mineral supplements to treat hypertension. Most of Kempner's patients experienced decreases in blood pressure as did patients treated by other investigators using similar diets. Presumably Kempner would have had better results by using brown rice rather than white rice and excluding sugar. World famous healer Alice J. Chase used a diet of raw fruit with bed rest to treat hypertension. She claims complete success with most patients within two weeks. Her most difficult cases required several weeks before "a change for the better" occurred. Middle aged men taking the SGA diet had systolic blood pressure drops to 110–120 millimeters.[207]

There is considerable epidemological data to support the effectiveness of more vegetarian salt-free diets in keeping blood pressure low. The New Guinea highlanders who experience declining blood pressure with age take no salt and rely almost exclusively on a single tuber for their "good health." The Abkhasians take what is very nearly a lacto-vegetarian salt-free diet. The Seventh Day Adventists who are urged to abstain from animal products and salt have much lower death rates from diseases associated with hypertension than do comparable non-Adventists. In a study unrelated to the Adventists, it was found the blood pressure of vegetarian monks was consistently lower than the pressure of meat-eating monks at every age. In their native land, Chinese rely on diets consisting primarily of grains and vegetables and avoid high blood pressure, but Chinese Americans who use quantities of salt and generally eat flesh every meal tend to have high blood pressure. There can scarcely be any doubt any group taking a salt-free vegan diet would be free from hypertension.[208]

The SGA diet meets every requirement for an ideal diet to effect and maintain low blood pressure. It is, first and foremost, a salt-free vegan regime. In addition, it contains rich supplies of potassium, calcium, magnesium and niacin. It is very low in fat and does not carry an excess of protein. Also important is the capacity of the SGA diet to prevent atherosclerosis which could lead to hypertension through damage to the kidneys. The SGA diet offers added protection to the kidneys by its buffering capacity, favorable calcium to phosphorus ratio and freedom from alcohol, coffee, tea and other stimulants as well as potentially toxic food additives.[209]

Not surprisingly, individuals who adopt the SGA diet invariably achieve very low blood pressure levels. This has not proved to be the case with the Kempner diet, and Chase noted only strict adherence to her whole-foods vegan diet would bring uniformly lower blood pressure levels. Evidently, dietary treatment of high blood pressure demands a greater degree of constraint than does the treatment of elevated serum cholesterol or triglycerides. But all things come of a carefully chosen vegan diet.[210]

OTHER FACTORS

Diabetics are highly vulnerable to atherosclerosis. Diabetes represents the extreme in elevated serum glucose (blood sugar) and glucose intolerance (abnormal rise in serum glucose after an intravenous or oral dose of glucose). Poor glucose tolerance has been found to raise the risk of coronary heart disease as much as high blood pressure or elevated serum cholesterol.[211]

Obesity raises the risk of all cardiovascular diseases. Obese persons were found to have an incidence of coronary heart disease double that of persons of normal weight. The death rate from strokes is evidently more than twice as high for obese individuals than nonobese individuals. To a considerable degree, obesity, like diabetes, is linked to impaired carbohydrate metabolism and both obesity and diabetes reflect similar metabolic abnormalities and origins. Obesity is strongly linked to hypertension also.[212]

Diabetes has been successfully treated with low-fat, sugar-free primarily vegetarian diets, and the Seventh Day Adventists have a mortality rate from diabetes about half that of others. Obesity has been most successfully treated with low-fat, high-carbohydrate diets. High fat and high protein intake along with the use of processed grains, sugar and salt tend to promote obesity. But eating only at meal times and taking fewer meals may aid in combating obesity. Vegetarian diets have been shown to lead to uniformly lower weights.[213]

It is important to remember that a diet designed to combat cardiovascular disease is also ideal for protection against diabetes and obesity. The only new finding is that eating less frequently might offer an advantage in controlling food intake. The SGA diet has proved to be very effective in lowering weight, and has resulted in no secondary complications such as losses of energy. Indeed individuals tend to become much more active on the SGA diet.[214]

Smoking is yet another factor which tends to raise the risk of cardiovascular disease. It was reported that the incidence of coronary heart disease in male patients at Mayo Clinic was three times as high for cigarette smokers as for nonsmokers. A study of Cincinnati residents found heavy smokers under 60 years old had a mortality rate from coronary heart disease double that of nonsmokers of the same age. Statistical analyst Cuglar Hammond offered the following relationship between coronary mortality rates and amounts of cigarettes smoked:[215]

Mortality from Coronaries
vs.
Amounts of Cigarettes Smoked

Coronary artery disease mortality ratio	Amount smoked per day
1.0	0
1.29	less than ½ pack
1.89	½ to 1 pack
2.15	1 to 2 packs
2.41	over 2 packs

It was found in the aforementioned Framingham study that smokers with elevated blood pressure and high serum cholesterol had an incidence of coronary heart disease ten times that of nonsmokers with normal serum cholesterol and blood pressure. Smoking evidently complicates hypertension, and there appears to be a substantial increase in the mortality rate from strokes among smokers. A recent report in the Wall Street Journal indicates smoking may increase the risk of strokes much more dramatically than was originally realized. A single inhalation of tobacco smoke tends to constrict the arteroles (smaller arteries at the surface of the skin) and may cause blood stoppage in the arteroles of the heart. However, the vascular constriction associated with smoking is not universal and the exact manner in which tobacco affects cardiovascular disease is unknown. But whatever the mechanism, smoking seems to be responsible for hundreds of thousands of cardiovascular fatalities each year and the cessation of smoking should be a national goal.[216]

There is evidence that the desire to smoke is related to diet: the Abkhasians raise tobacco, but in spite of its ready availability, they rarely smoke; only 7% of a group of British vegans were smokers while over 70% of nonvegetarian Britians smoked. Whole-foods diets free from coffee and other stimulants may have aided many Mormons and Seventh Day Adventists to give up smoking.[217]

Smoking tends to be associated with reliance on other forms of stimulation including caffeine, sugar, salt, vitamin pills, medicines and other drugs as well as alcohol and possibly meat. The relationship between smoking and sugar intake has been verified by British researchers. Milder diets are bound to reduce the need to smoke.[218]

Arguments that atherosclerosis is brought about by "emotional stress" have been largely discredited. Dr. Paul Dudley White says flatly that disturbed emotions do not cause heart disease, and it has been noted that groups subjected to the rigors of war and kept in states of semistarvation have experienced low incidences of coronary heart disease. During the second World War, the Germans occupied Norway subjecting Norwegians to "great nervous strain and anxiety" and to food scarcity, particularly for meat and dairy products. During the occupation, the death rate from coronary heart disease fell by a third in the cities and by 22% in the less affected rural areas.[219]

Certainly if stress were a killer, it would play havoc with America's top executives. But Metropolitan Life Insurance Company has found the Board Chairmen of the nation's 500 largest corporations have a death rate 31% lower than average for men their age. If Board chairmen are above the daily stresses of business, Presidents of corporations are less likely to be so: Metropolitan found the death rate for Presidents of the 500 biggest corporations was 42% below average for their age. Capacity for work is impaired by dietary excesses, and many executives may use restraint at meals to keep themselves working efficiently. The demands on corporate leaders are physical as well as psychological and to the extent stress is demanding physically, it may actually stave off cardiovascular disease. Exercise reduced the build-up of atherosclerosis in pigs fed fat and cholesterol and rigorous physical training tends to lower serum cholesterol and triglycerides in men.[220]

DIETARY CHANGES

In less orthodox ways, young Americans are turning to vegetarianism in growing numbers. The movement, if with its diverse nature it can be called a movement, was first seen at the fringes of University communities and in cultural centers. It has now reached the stage of being openly recommended in classrooms and is widespread in rural areas where large scale agriculture is limited. If the entire U.S. population were to switch to vegan diets, grains now used to fatten animals could be diverted to human use and a billion or more of the world's hungry could be fed. Thus vegetarianism is a moral issue involving more than animals: we eat a steak at the expense of forcing thirty people to do without a meal.[221]

Judging from the emergence of opposition to the Vietnam War and the quest for civil equality, just causes begin on a small scale in the United States, but aided by press and television coverage such causes can change a nation. Currently, the media is confronting us with grim statistics about the "World Food Crises" and the woes of life in Bangladesh, Central Africa and populous India. "Tell them to take birth control pills" is not a reasoned response to the situation. To be sure, family size must be limited but even when a Bangladesh couple limits their offspring to two, or one, or *none*, we ignore their hunger. The hard facts of our callousness are not news to the rest of the world, and they can become the rallying point for environmentalists, consumer advocates, spiritual and religious reformers, conservationists, human rights proponents, etc. The path to simplicity and its deep rewards will not be without pitfalls, of course.[222]

Food processors view the need for cutting intake of meat, eggs, dairy products, sugar and salt and boosting vitamin R intake as an opportunity to fatten themselves economically. Giving no mention to their past and present roles in actively promoting the use of the very products that need replacement, the processing giants now plan to peddle such engineering marvels as artificial hot dogs, meatless steaks (with plastic T-bones perhaps?), simulated milk, artificial sweeteners, etc. If the processors get their way they will have 200 million (actively solicited) volunteers for an experiment on the long term effects of a semisynthetic diet on man. We know our first brushes with semisynthetic foods (e.g. refined grains and sugar) are disastrous, and we know laboratory animals have greater incidences of atherosclerosis, cancer, obesity, etc. and have shorter life spans on semisynthetic diets. On the other hand if semisynthetic foods were taken off the food counters certain big companies might be at a loss to remain very big companies.[223]

The food processors seem quite confident the public will turn to them for their new food needs. At the annual meeting of the Institute of Food Technologists in 1973, it was asserted that only "highly motivated" individuals will be satisfied with "cereal products" in lieu of red meat. There is considerably more to a vegan diet than "cereal products," of course, and the way to get people "highly motivated" to partake of whole-foods (i.e. unprocessed) vegan diets is to tell them the truth, rather than scheming for sales of today's remedy (and tomorrow's cause) for yesterday's innovations.[224]

The truth is that degenerative disease afflicts most Americans by early childhood and seemingly all Americans (taking the normal U.S. diet) by early adulthood. The truth is almost all Americans die of degenerative disease: the "lucky" ones go from sudden, unexpected heart attacks or strokes; others are given veritable death sentences by surviving a stroke or heart attack; still others watch while diabetes, osteoporosis or multiple sclerosis slowly eradicate their being. Others suffer the horrors of cancer. The truth is none of these diseases are necessary, and there is every reason to believe these maladies are self-inflicted. The truth is our eating, drinking and smoking habits have been directly implicated in every major form of degenerative disease.

The truth is that meat, eggs, dairy products and fats and oils head the list of ill-chosen food items. The truth is sugar, salt and refined grains are willing accomplices, if not equal partners, in the path to degeneration. The truth is alcohol, coffee and such standbys as aspirin, are all implicated in major degenerative diseases. The truth is smoking affects a lot more than emphysema and lung cancer though the latter is sufficient to classify cigarettes as deadly. The truth is no scientific miracle is going to correct greed and over-indulgence; no pills or powders will prepare the intestines or liver or kidneys for the onslaught of excesses and toxins in today's, much less what technologists picture as tomorrow's diet.[225]

Some of these truths are apparent from the previous discussion of cardiovascular disease. The other assertions are expanded and corroborated in subsequent sections of this book. The immediate question is to what degree can and will Americans change their way of eating. Even the food processors look for big reductions in intake of beef, pork, eggs, cheese, whole milk, lamb, sugar and salt, and very limited intake of cholesterol-rich organ meats. These certainly represent major changes to most individuals and the motivation is based on nothing more than an expected decrease in incidence of coronary heart disease. How much greater the motivation to change would be if a new diet combined with a cessation of smoking could be expected to bring an *end* to coronary heart disease . . . and strokes . . . and hypertension . . . and atherosclerosis . . . and diabetes . . . and multiple sclerosis . . . and ulcers . . . and obesity . . . and hypoglycemia . . . and tooth decay . . . and the disabilities of aging . . . and cancer . . . and many, if not all, emotional disorders. The SGA diet is such a regime and after a switch to the SGA diet, the task of giving up smoking has proved to be no task at all.[226]

Judging by the effect of less promising vegan diets on serum cholesterol and the effect of sugar-free vegan diets on serum triglycerides, a switch to an SGA-type diet should result in a serum cholesterol level of under 200 milligrams percent and serum triglyceride levels of less than 100 milligrams percent. Heart attacks are very rare with such readings, and there is every reason to believe the SGA diet would prevent atherosclerosis completely if begun early enough. Judging by the experience of the Abkhasians even a sound whole-foods, lacto-vegetarian diet should offer strong protection against atherosclerosis. A primarily vegetarian diet which included seafood on occasion might also thwart atherosclerosis.[227]

It is often argued that Americans simply will not change their way of eating, and even if they did there is no irrefutable evidence they would be better off. Countering these claims are a number of observations including the practices of the Seventh Day Adventists. Thanks to research at Loma Linda University and the urgings of a few reform-minded leaders, half of the world's two million Adventists now voluntarily adhere to vegetarian diets. Their rewards include much lower death rates from all the major killers, including not only coronary heart disease and strokes but cancer, diabetes, ulcers, lung disorders, automobile accidents and even suicide. It is easy to dismiss the Adventists' willingness to change by claiming vegetarianism is part of their religion but this is not strictly true. In the eyes of the Adventists, vegetarianism is not a condition for salvation, membership in the Church or even Church leadership.[228]

Completely divorced from religion is the Kempner "rice diet" which is completely free of animal products. In spite of its very high content of refined carbohydrates, especially sugar, the Kempner diet has resulted in weight loss along with reductions in blood pressure and serum cholesterol for most individuals who have tried the regime. If Americans were unwilling to make major changes in their way of eating, they certainly would have nothing to do with the Kempner diet but would-be rice-dieters became so numerous that they were forced to wait for months for available clinic space to participate in the Kempner program.[229]

The results of long term studies on the effect of specific dietary changes on the incidence of coronary heart disease shows reductions in meat, eggs and sugar can save lives and that individuals can and do adapt to the changes.[230]

Typical is the experience of the New York Anticoronary Club where volunteers who had no history of heart disease were put on a diet restricting their intake of beef, mutton and pork to four or less small servings per week. They were urged to avoid eggs, butter, cheeses and pastries. Fish and seafoods were recommended as regular items and skimmed milk was suggested as a replacement for whole milk. Very few of those with normal weight dropped out of the experiment, but 30% or more of those who were overweight, and who were asked to cut their caloric intake in half and reduce their fat intake by 90% did drop out.[231]

The New York Anticoronary Club members began their modified diet with an average cholesterol level of 260 milligrams percent. In one year, the average had fallen to 230 milligrams percent and it fell an additional 5 milligrams percent each year for the next four years. Thus, based on serum cholesterol levels, the Club as a whole went from a high risk category to a low risk category. After the first year, the incidence of coronary heart disease was 0.34% per year for Club members and 0.98% for comparable individuals taking normal diets. These results suggest a nationwide effort to cut egg, meat and free fat intake could prevent hundreds of thousands of heart attacks per year.[232]

An earlier study in Chicago centered on men 40 to 59 years of age who were regarded as high risks. The subjects were urged to avoid egg yolks, fatty meats, ice cream, butter and most cheeses. They were urged to take fruits, nuts, vegetables and legumes along with fish, seafood and poultry. About a third of those who started the program dropped out during the first two years but few left the program thereafter. Cholesterol levels fell an average of 15% in the first few weeks and very few appeared to be resistant to the lowering effect of the dietary changes.[233]

Similar studies have been done with volunteers in Los Angeles and diabetic patients in Iowa City. A 12-year study carried out at two Helsinki hospitals pointed to the importance of cutting sugar intake to reduce the incidence of coronary heart disease. In a ten-year study in Montclair, New Jersey, 100 men with confirmed coronary artery disease and previous heart attacks were put on a diet containing 28% fat with less than one third of their fat saturated and with their cholesterol intake cut in half. Sixteen members of the experimental group suffered fatal heart attacks during the ten-year span. Twenty-eight members of a control group died from heart attacks, and the results were much more impressive for those who made the dietary changes before age 45.[234]

While all the long term studies of the effects of less animal-oriented diets have yielded impressive reductions in mortality from coronaries, they have not brought about significant reductions in deaths from cancer or even strokes. However, there probably would have been a sharp drop in cancer mortality if refined grains and stimulants had been eliminated from the experimental diets. The Mormons have an incidence of cancer some 40% below that of individuals living and eating in the normal American way. They do not smoke and "practice moderation in the eating of meat" while emphasizing the use of unrefined grains and fresh fruits and vegetables. Judging by the experience of the Seventh Day Adventists, even sharper drops in the incidence of cancer plus big reductions in the incidence of strokes, diabetes and other degenerative disease would have been evident if meat had been eliminated entirely.[235]

In the past, researchers have replaced animal fats with polyunsaturated vegetable fats in anticoronary diets to a degree that has left the diets very high (28% or more of calories) in total fat. High fat intake has been implicated in more degenerative diseases than any other dietary factor. It is strongly implicated in cancer of the uterus, cancer of the breast, cancer of the rectum, cancer of the colon, cancer of the pancreas, cancer of the gall bladder, multiple sclerosis, diabetes, obesity, strokes, arthritis, leukemia and reduced life span. With a decline in coronary heart disease, individuals might be expected to experience an increase in some other degenerative diseases, albeit at later ages. A diet aimed at ending rather than reducing coronaries would have required sharply cutting fat levels as well as curtailing processed foods and such changes should effect reductions in virtually all the major degenerative diseases. In the past, experimental diets all but ignored hypertension (high blood pressure) which greatly elevates the risk of coronaries and strokes, and of itself, constitutes a major cardiovascular disease. But preventing high blood pressure would have meant offering foods with satisfying tastes of their own rather than products requiring salt and that would indeed have been a radical change.[236]

SUMMARY:

Atherosclerosis is believed to fester in the arteries of every adult taking standard Western diets. Rising serum cholesterol and/or triglycerides are normative in North America, and they announce an advanced state of atherosclerosis and increasing risk of a seizure. The principle causes of the condition are dietary cholesterol and fat, especially saturated fat. All of the cholesterol and virtually all of the saturated fat is derived from animal products (meat, eggs, dairy products, etc.). The U.S. diet is sickeningly high in sugar which tends to cause dramatic increases in serum triglycerides.[237]

Practically everything in the U.S. diet which does not contain sugar is given a dousing with salt, which tends to elevate blood pressure, thus boosting the risk of seizures. Virtually all of the grains in the normal U.S. diet are refined, hence very low in (serum cholesterol lowering) vitamin R. Caffeine, alcohol, drugs (including medicines) and even chlorinated tap water may play important roles in atherosclerosis also. While atherosclerosis is basically a disease of excesses of animal products and refined foods, it may be exacerbated by low levels of several vitamins and minerals which tend to be in short supply in the normal U.S. diet.[238]

Individuals taking more vegetarian diets tend to maintain low serum cholesterol levels and to avoid atherosclerosis. Vegan diets result in sharp reductions in serum cholesterol in humans and regressions in atherosclerosis in animals. The effectiveness of a vegan diet is enhanced by the absence of processed foods, especially sugar, which strongly influences serum triglyceride levels.[239]

The SGA diet (which consists of large quantities of raw sprouts and soybeans, legumes and grains, raw, dark green leafy vegetables, with a smattering of seaweed, plus baked tubers and fruit) is exceptionally low in total fat, even compared to other vegan diets; it contains no processed foods and it is free of salt, other stimulants and questionable chlorinated water. In addition, the SGA diet is unmatched for its rich content of vitamins and minerals including those tending to prevent atherosclerosis.[240]

Hypertension (high blood pressure) which aggravates atherosclerosis and constitutes a major cardiovascular disease in itself is closely linked to excessive salt intake. Salt-free vegetarian diets tend to result in low blood pressure while the normal U.S. diet leads to rising blood pressure with age. A whole-foods, salt-free vegan diet has brought reductions in blood pressure to even the most severe cases of hypertension but lesser dietary changes have not been totally effective.[241]

The SGA diet offers ideal protection against high blood pressure: it is not only a salt-free, whole-foods vegan regime but offers rich quantities of nutrients which aid in protection against hypertension,

and it is exceptionally low in substances which may aid salt in boosting blood pressure. In practice, the SGA diet has brought uniformly
favorable blood pressure levels.[242]

Other factors tending to affect the risk of cardiovascular disease
include impaired carbohydrate metabolism, obesity and smoking.
Whole-foods, low-fat vegan diets (e.g. the SGA diet) have precisely
the properties necessary to end obesity and to avoid, and quite possibly cure, even advanced cases of impaired carbohydrate metabolism. There may be some advantage in eating fewer times each day
and there is evidence that whole-foods vegan diets can aid in bringing
an end to smoking also. Thus, carefully constructed whole-foods
vegan diets such as the SGA diet tend to thwart the development of
cardiovascular disease on every front.[243]

The AMA and National Research Council have recognized the
need to change the U.S. diet in order to reduce the incidence of coronary heart disease. To this end, they have made recommendations,
but the result of their plan may be an even more highly processed
diet, and quite possibly, an increase in the number of individuals suc-
cumbing to strokes and cancer. With a switch to the SGA diet, however, the nation could expect an end (rather than simply a reduction)
to coronary heart disease. Even more important is the fact that all
cardiovascular disease, and indeed all degenerative disease should
vanish with the adoption of the SGA diet.[244]

3 / diseases related to carbohydrate metabolism:
diabetes, obesity, emotional disorders, multiple sclerosis and cystic fibrosis

Cancer, cardiovascular disorders and other degenerative diseases are beginning to be recognized not so much as separate entities, but as different manifestations of a handful of basic underlying conditions. In the future we may see cancer, diabetes and even atherosclerosis classified as liver disorders. Or we may see cancer, muscular dystrophy, obesity, gout and osteoporosis classified as manifestations of excesses of dietary protein or "protein foods." Diabetes, cystic fibrosis and hypoglycemia may come to be recognized as pancreatic disorders or fat and sugar maladies, etc.[245]

The present chapter is concerned with diseases related to disturbances in carbohydrate metabolism; the chapter deals for the most part with conditions associated with abnormalities in blood sugar levels. Contrary to contemporary folklore such diseases are not caused by an excess of carbohydrates. Indeed carbohydrate-rich *whole-foods* tend to protect against such diseases; it is excesses of refined carbohydrates, especially sugar, that implicate carbohydrates in such disorders. By way of contrast *all fats have been implicated in conditions related to carbohydrate metabolism*. Deficiencies are also involved.[246]

Low blood sugar tends to starve the brain and nervous system which results in degeneration of nervous tissues and emotional disorders ranging from schizophrenia to paranoia and from irritability to lassitude. The degradation of nerve tissue may also take the form of multiple sclerosis. High blood sugar is the principle symptom of diabetes, which affects the liver and pancreas. Closely related to, and often combined with, diabetes is obesity; and cystic fibrosis like diabetes, is related to pancreatic insufficiency.[247]

As a rule diseases related to disturbed carbohydrate metabolism do not kill quickly. Rather they bring the victim down slowly and irregularly over a period of years. Conventional medicine offers no cures simply because it fails to deal with the cause: food. A carefully chosen diet offers complete protection against impaired carbohydrate metabolism, and it can serve as a complete cure for related diseases if it is initiated in the early stages of the disorders.[248]

DIABETES

Diabetes is a disease in which blood sugar (serum glucose) concentrations become so pronounced that glucose is passed in the urine. The ingestion of food causes a temporary increase in serum glucose concentrations which then proceed to return to normal fasting levels. (Hereafter the term "fasting" is used in the sense of the clinical definition of "not in the act of consuming food.") Impaired carbohydrate metabolism is evidenced by differences from the norm in fasting serum glucose levels and/or exceptionally large increases in serum glucose following ingestion (or intravenous feeding) of pure glucose. Glucose (or a "glucose load") is used to gauge transient response to food simply as a matter of convenience; exceptionally large and prolonged increases in serum glucose in response to a glucose load is called impaired glucose tolerance or just glucose intolerance.[249]

Diabetes represents the pathological extremes in glucose intolerance and elevated fasting glucose levels. The latter results from failure of body cells to utilize serum glucose so that glucose accumulates in the blood. Insulin, a hormone which is produced by the pancreas, stimulates body cells to take up glucose for energy and the liver to take up glucose for storage. In diabetes, either the pancreatic synthesis of insulin is decreased or the cells of the body and the liver fail to respond to the presence of normal concentrations of insulin. Fat metabolism is also impaired in diabetes; the rate of fatty acid synthesis is decreased and the utilization of fatty acids for energy is accelerated. The rate of tissue protein breakdown may also be accelerated.[250]

Diabetics are spared quick death by regular injections of synthetic insulin, or insulin take from animals, but even with the injections, their lives remain "short and trouble." When a child develops diabetes, his or her life expectancy is cut to less than 30 years; adult diabetics also experience drastic reductions in life expectancy. Atherosclerosis tends to afflict diabetics at very young ages. As a result, diabetics are highly prone to strokes, and studies in Sweden, Britain and the U.S. show the risk of coronaries rises sharply with increasing glucose intolerance. Arterial degeneration often affects the eyes, nerves and kidneys of diabetics: the disease is now the leading cause of new cases of blindness in the U.S. and many diabetics dies from kidney failure while others undergo amputations for gangrene. Impotence and pregnancy problems are common among diabetics also.[251]

Impaired carbohydrate metabolism may be involved in various cancers and pancreatic cancer has been linked directly to diabetes. Diabetes itself takes some 20,000 lives per year and complications arising from diabetes have led the president of the American Diabetes Association to label diabetes "the United States' second leading cause of death."[252]

There are about 6 million known diabetics in the U.S. today and the number is doubling every 12 years. The number of potential diabetics is staggering: studies of 2000 seemingly healthy Muscovites in their 50's and 3000 hospital patients in Chicago showed about half of each group suffered from impaired glucose tolerance. And an insulin test of the 1500 Chicago patients with no signs of glucose intolerance showed half of that group had "diabetic patterns." These findings suggest the food-rich nations may be headed for a state in which still another pathological condition will become "normal."[253]

Population studies on the incidences of diabetes are somewhat limited, but when natives of India migrate to South Africa or rural South Africans migrate to urban areas, a sharp increase in the incidence of diabetes occurs. The moves lead to marked increases in sugar intake. After 20 years in Israel, Yemenites experienced a thirtyfold greater prevalence of diabetes than new arrivals from Yemen. On a worldwide basis, there is a strong correlation between sugar intake and deaths due to diabetes. On the other hand, it is reported that the incidence of human diabetes is correlated with the amount of fat consumed. These are not conflicting findings; rather they are two aspects of the same problem.[254]

Sugar tends to impair the functions of both the pancreas and the liver. When rats are fed high-sugar levels over a prolonged period, their pancreases show declining ability to produce insulin and their livers tend to weaken and swell. Rats were found to contract impaired glucose tolerance after only three months on diets containing average U.S. sugar levels, and when their sugar level was doubled, the impairment developed in only three weeks. High levels of sugar tend to reduce the ability of the liver and body cells to take up and utilize glucose. The eyes of rats on high-sugar diets show a tendency to degenerate in a manner that is often seen in severe human diabetes and kidney failure, which is common among human diabetics, and can also be induced in rats by feeding them diets high in sugar. On the other hand, high-starch diets tend to protect rats against impaired glucose tolerance, pancreatic damage, liver dysfunction, eye damage and kidney failure. Rats are not spared these afflictions by a switch from white sugar to brown sugar or the addition of chromium to sugar in their diets.[255]

In a study comparing the effects of sugar and starch on carbohydrate metabolism in humans, eight "healthy" adults were fed five weeks on sugar-free diets in which 60% of calories were supplied by bread. Seven other adults took at least four ounces of sugar per day and then the diets of the two groups were reversed for five weeks. The peak serum glucose reading after an oral glucose load averaged 180 milligrams per 100 milliliters with sugar compared to 125 milligrams per 100 milliliters with starch in the form of bread. In a British study, nine middle-aged subjects had lower fasting serum glucose when most of their carbohydrate consisted of starch than when most of their carbohydrate was taken as sugar.[256]

While starch is far superior to sugar in building defenses against impaired carbohydrate metabolism, whole foods, rich in starch, tend to be considerably more effective than refined grains or starch extracts. Refined starches have been found to cause "diabetic symptoms" in mice, and the tendency of refined starches to elevate serum triglycerides suggests they affect carbohydrate metabolism in much the same way as sugar.[257]

In the short run, all forms of carbohydrate tend to promote lower serum glucose and lessen the rise in serum glucose following a glucose load. But sugar achieves the reductions at the expense of an increase in serum insulin. Elevated serum insulin is an acknowledged pre-diabetic condition which is believed to result from over stimulation of the pancreas. In time, the repeated overstimulation of the pancreas by sugar tends to result in pathologically low levels or diabetically high levels of serum glucose; in either case, response to a glucose load tends to be impaired. The favorable effect of starch-rich foods on serum glucose shows no tendency to deteriorate with time.[258]

The role of sugar in diabetes is well recognized, but the standard U.S. diet for diabetes fails to take into account the ability of starch-rich foods to improve glucose tolerance. U.S. diabetics are advised to avoid all carbohydrates and are given high-fat diets rich in meat and other animal products. High-fat intake tends to tax the liver and fatty livers are strongly associated with diabetes in humans. Japanese researchers have found high-fat diets induce impaired glucose tolerance and decrease insulin sensitivity in rats, and it has been suggested the tendency to replace dietary carbohydrates with fat is a contributing factor in human diabetes.[259]

The role of fat in diabetes implicates animal products in the disease but fat may not be the only diabetic factor in animal products. Tests showed defatted egg worked with sugar to cause a (prediabetic) rise in serum insulin in rats and an excess of methionine (in which the protein of eggs, meat, fish and milk are high) impaired the glucose tolerance of rats.[260]

The standard Japanese diet for diabetics is low in fat and animal products and high in carbohydrate (as refined rice), and the Japanese diet has proved far more successful than the U.S. diet for diabetics. The Japanese regime has led not only to a lower death rate from diabetes as such, but has resulted in dramatic reductions in cardiovascular complications associated with diabetes. Studies showed only one in twenty Japanese diabetics died from coronary heart disease while eleven out of every twenty American diabetics succumbed to coronaries. U.S. practitioners who employ food to treat disease are well aware of the need to keep fat intake low, but low-fat diets are not used by the establishment because they "would require major adjustments."[261]

The life of a diabetic requires unprecedented adjustments and risks any concerned person would like to avoid. There is little hope of avoiding the "major adjustments" of blindness, loss of limbs, atherosclerosis and early death with the standard U.S. diet for diabetics, but there is strong hope for diabetics who are willing to switch to the whole-foods, low-fat, sugar-free carbohydrate diets.[262]

In a magnificent break with established practices, an Indian physician, Dr. Inder Singh, restricted 80 diabetic patients to 20 to 30 grams of fat per day and forbade their taking sugar. In three to six weeks 50 of the Indian physicians' 80 patients required no more insulin. In the weeks that followed eight more were freed of insulin and most of the remaining patients had their insulin needs cut to a small fraction of their original levels. All 80 cases were monitored for periods ranging from six months to five years. One patient who returned to a high-fat diet after one year regained her high fasting glucose level and poor glucose tolerance status. But after a two-week return to the low-fat diet she was again "cured."[263]

Singh's remarkable success stands in contrast to the failure of patients to escape the use of insulin with the Japanese diabetic diet which is also high in starch and low in fat. On the other hand, the Indian staple is whole wheat, usually taken as chappaties, whereas the Japanese diet is dominated by white (i.e. refined) rice. There is no record of exactly what Singh's patients did eat since he treated them on an out-patient basis. The failure of about 10% of his patients to respond to his dietary regime may well have been due to their using white flour, which he did not forbid, or even fat and sugar, if clandestinely.[264]

As a result of the work by Singh and others, Indian diabetics are now usually advised of the possibility of avoiding drug-dependence by adherence to a low-fat diet which is free of refined carbohydrates. It is estimated that about half of the patients so advised opt for the dietary change, and almost all of those remain symptom-free.[265]

The failure of U.S. physicians to utilize low-fat diets in treating diabetics is difficult to understand. The excuse that such a diet would require "major adjustments" is untenable: only the diabetic who everyday faces an ebbing struggle for his very existence can say whether he is willing to change. And he deserves the opportunity to make the decision. What he doesn't deserve is rhetoric about the lack of necessary nutrients in vegan diets (for indeed a diet containing 20 to 30 grams of fat would of necessity be free of meat, eggs, cheese, whole milk, fish, etc.). By taking a raw-foods diet rich in grain sprouts and bean sprouts, and dark green leafy vegetables such as collards, parsley, turnip greens and watercress and including a little seaweed, one can obtain abundant amounts of every necessary nutrient. To the sprouts, greens and seaweed could be added Irish potatoes but diabetics should avoid fruit, at least until insulin is no longer needed. The initial diet is, in effect, a (literally) fruitless version of the SGA diet. It must be made clear though, that improvement depends on a permanent change. Singh's work shows clearly that staying off of insulin injections requires staying on the diet which allowed the break.[266]

For those who have not yet reached the state of clinical diabetes, there is the promise of complete freedom from impaired carbohydrate metabolism by a change to a low-fat, sugar-free, starch-rich, whole-foods diet. And from recent studies, it appears the risk of impaired carbohydrate metabolism or diabetic findings is becoming the risk of reaching 60 years of age . . . or is it 30 years?[267]

OBESITY

Closely related to diabetes is obesity. In one clinical study it was noted diabetic and obese individuals exhibited common hormonal and metabolic abnormalities; in another study, it was found 94 of 100 obese children had impaired carbohydrate metabolism. Many, if not most, diabetics are obese and one researcher reported there is strong evidence excessive food intake and inactivity are responsible for liver dysfunction in diabetes.[268]

Obesity is recognized by an overweight condition, but the term actually refers to the deposition of excess body fat. Nonobese adults normally have less than 15 kilograms of body fat, but obese individuals often carry 60 kilograms of fat or more. Fat tissue constitutes up to half of the body weight of obese persons but fat accounts for only about 20% of the body weight of normal individuals. Obesity is thus very accurately described as "being fat." Moderate obesity has been associated with an increase in the number of adipose (fat) cells, while severe obesity is believed to result primarily in an increase in the size of adipose cells.[269]

Obesity is more than an eyesore. There is a large and consistent body of data indicating obesity "even to a mild degree" results in higher incidences of heart and circulatory diseases, diabetes, liver disorders, gall bladder disease, arthritis and numerous other degenerative diseases. Earlier it was shown obesity raised the risk of cancer markedly, and a German medical-research team is said to have found there is a very high incidence of infant mortality among the offspring of obese mothers. There is a marked drop in longevity in obesity: according to one assessment an obese teenager has a life expectancy 15 years less than normal. On the other hand, a teenager who remains 20% under the normal weight enjoys a 15 year increase over and above normal life expectancy. Lower than normal weight is also associated with marked reductions in the incidence of cancer, cardiovascular diseases, diabetes and other degenerative diseases. In a very real sense then, U.S. and European weight standards are excessive, and the overwhelming majority of Americans and Europeans are detrimentally overweight, if not clinically obese.[270]

In one survey of professional men and their wives four in ten admitted to being overweight, and the U.S. Public Health Service estimates 60 million Americans are overweight. In reality the number of Americans who are above optimal weight may be three times the government estimate. A study of German industrial workers showed 41% of the males and 66% of the females were overweight while a survey of over 2500 persons of school age and beyond in rural Poland showed over 25% were overweight. These figures, especially the German ones, are alarming at face value, but when the likelihood that the norms are excessive is taken into account, it depicts Northern Europe as a veritable feed lot.[271]

Obesity is obviously a major problem in the heavy meat-eating nations of the West, but it is rare in rural areas of India, China, Indo-China and Africa where diets are very low in animal products. The essentially lacto-vegetarian Abkhasians remain "slim but strong" into very advanced ages and the almost totally vegetarian Hunzas were never seen to be overweight. Ethiopian villagers on an essentially vegan diet were found to take only about half as many calories as Westerners and the lesser intakes were of the villagers choosing, rather than of necessity.[272]

An Argentine study indicated obesity was a severe problem where meat-eating is encouraged, and a number of studies have shown American and European vegetarians weigh less than meat-eaters. It has been further shown that vegans tend to weigh considerably less than lacto-vegetarians. One researcher summarized his observations by saying a strict vegetarian diet gives individuals a slim, under-weight (meaning under normal weight) body.[273]

Dr. Henry Bieler, author of *Food is Your Best Medicine*, proceeded to take his patients off of meat as a first step in treating obesity, and Dr. Alice Chase had her obese patients alternate between fasting and a diet of freshly made fruit and vegetable juices, salads and fruits. Initially she had them stay in bed but in time she advised them to do some exercises consisting of alternately tensing and relaxing "every muscle of the body." After 23 years experience with the treatment, she reported that in every case where patients cooperate, success in reducing weight to normal as well as maintaining it at a normal level is obtained. She advised a diet of raw fruits, raw vegetables, "properly cooked" vegetables and dairy products for the maintenance of good health.[274]

The SGA diet has brought a rapid end to obesity in individuals of various ages and a transient weakness which seems to have ac-companied the treatments of Bieler and Chase has not been seen with the SGA regime. A 52 year-old man became weak during a mild case of diarrhea which lasted for one day some two months after beginning the SGA diet but no other difficulties, transitional or otherwise, have been seen. The individual in question had a drop in weight from over 200 pounds to under 170 pounds after about 4½ months on the SGA diet. His weight eventually stabilized at about 168 pounds which is close to optimal for his six-foot, one-inch height.[275]

The problem of obesity among individuals taking the usual Amer-ican diet evidently results primarily from an excess of fat in conjunc-tion with a high level of protein in their diets. Refined foods, especially sugar, may also play an important role in the obesity prob-lem. Salt, beverages containing caffeine and eating between meals may likewise be involved. Vegetarians, especially vegans, have been found to take less fat and less protein than meat-eaters and they tend to avoid refined foods, salt and coffee. It is not surprising then that they are not bothered with obesity.[276]

There is strong evidence dietary fat plays a key role in obesity. Fat intake is high in all nations where obesity is a major problem, and obesity is rare in countries in which fat intake is very limited. More-over, low-fat diets, especially high-carbohydrate diets, are very effective in treating obesity. Research with animals leaves no doubt that high-fat intake, if complemented with an adequate supply of protein, can cause gross obesity. Animal fats (butter, tallow, lard, etc.) tend to produce the most severe states of obesity.[277]

Diets containing large amounts of butter cause extreme obesity in animals and successive generations of rats fed butter-rich diets suffered from fatty livers and other disturbances related to obesity as well as obesity itself. Vegetable oils have been found to cause lesser degrees of obesity than animal fats, but all fats tend to produce gross excesses of body fat in animals. Laboratory tests have shown that even when the total caloric intake of animals taking high-fat diets does not exceed the caloric levels of grain-fed animals, the fat-eaters still tend to become obese.[278]

British scientists found rats had a significant increase in body fat after only 22 days on high-fat diets, and a leading researcher concluded from studies with mice that "the more fat in the diet the higher is the body fat content." Added vitamin intake seems to be no help in overcoming fat-induced obesity. In fact vitamin supplements tend to raise the degree of obesity in animals fed high-fat diets.[279]

Up until 1955, there were few animal studies to verify the role of dietary fat in obesity. Researchers now believe earlier attempts to promote obesity with high-fat diets failed simply because the fat was not combined with adequate quantities of protein. Investigators at the National Institute of Health used protein and fat levels equal to those of raw sirloin steak or ham to effect a doubling of the weight of rats from normal.[280]

The protein content of adipose tissue of obese mice proved to be significantly higher than that of nonobese mice, and it was found that food intake of rats taking high levels of protein had to be restricted in order to keep them from gaining more weight than rats taking lesser amounts of protein. Two British researchers found high-protein alone were more inclined to produce obesity in rats than high-fat alone. Predictably though, the combination of high-fat and high-protein yielded the greatest weight gains.[281]

Obese persons are often encouraged to become active physically, but Harvard's Dr. Gene Mayer noted that obese individuals have "startling differences" in energy output. He reported that even when playing tennis, obese persons exert themselves much less than normal individuals. Researchers have found obese individuals spend more time in bed and less time on their feet when not in bed than persons of normal weight. In theory caloric needs depend on body size but so slowed down were obese women that they burned no more calories than women weighing half as much. Other clinical findings have verified that as the degree of obesity increases physical activity decreases.[282]

Evidently the physical limit of obesity involves a state of total immobility. Between this limit and capacity for continuous physical activity are varying levels of physical endurance. Viewed in this way, obesity is associated with a very low level of endurance which suggests obesity might be treated by building the endurance of obese persons. While this reasoning borders on pure speculation, it is supported by the findings that diets that promote obesity hinder endurance while diets that bring weight losses enhance endurance.[283]

High-fat and/or high-protein diets which have been strongly implicated in obesity cause marked reductions in the endurance and spontaneous activity levels of laboratory animals. Researchers who study the relationship between diet and endurance recommend high carbohydrate diets for athletes in training. High carbohydrate diets have been shown to result in greater endurance in humans riding bicycle ergmeters and preparing for International athletic contests. Carbohydrates are recognized as the preferred energy source for working muscles. There is no increase in the need for protein (or fat) during heavy exercise even when it continues into exhaustion. Indeed high-fat, high-protein (meat based) diets have been shown to impair the performance of distance runners and cross-country skiers. The normal American diet contains three times as much protein and ten times as much fat as would benefit athletes seeking to better their performance.[284]

Endurance is not an innate characteristic: it must be established and nurtured. A high-carbohydrate diet tends to boost endurance and increase spontaneous activity, but these characteristics will continue only so long as the diet continues. A high-carbohydrate diet will also overcome obesity, but again lasting results depend on tenacity. It has resulted in a society which is almost universally overweight and which avoids any semblance of sustained activity.[285]

Chase and Bieler both offered obese patients low-fat, low-protein diets and had consistently favorable response to their treatments. The University of Oregon's Dr. R. L. Swank treated 146 multiple sclerosis patients with low-fat, high-carbohydrate diets and found their weight fell until it stabilized 5% to 10% under normal.[286]

The Kempner diet, which is very low in protein and fat and very high in carbohydrates (as rice and sugar) usually causes a substantial loss in weight, even when calories are unrestricted. A decade before the Kempner regime came into use, a Scandinavian researcher, Dr. Eggert Møller obtained excellent results by treating obesity with a low-protein, low-calorie diet. Dr. Vincent P. Dole and his colleagues at the Rockefeller Institute had remarkable success in treating obesity with a low-protein, high-carbohydrate diet. In the Dole study 36 obese individuals were offered a calorically unrestricted diet which contained only 35 grams protein per day with unlimited amounts of sugar, butter, coffee and tea. The subjects lost an average of over two pounds per week and 31 of the 36 lost a pound per week or more. None of the subjects gained weight; liver functions remained normal and the general health of all subjects remained good. Although their caloric and butter intakes were not restricted, the subjects took relatively little fat and far fewer calories than normal on their primarily vegetarian regime.[287]

Unfortunately Americans have been schooled to always look for a "cure," something they can take or undertake for a (hopefully brief) period to alleviate their health problems. A diet emphasizing lean meat and consisting almost entirely of animal products has brought temporary weight losses to many Americans, but recent studies at the University of Wisconsin and Peter Bent Brigham Hospital in Boston show even short periods on high-meat diets lead to devastating bone degeneration and dramatic rises in serum cholesterol levels. In the worst sense, high-meat diets are "crash diets."[288]

While crash diets are the usual vehicle for do-it-yourself weight watchers current medical treatment for obesity appears to be no less short-sighted. It is the vogue to put obese patients in hospitals where they are given very low-calorie diets or put on prolonged fasts until they have brought their weight into line or given up. Those who endure the hospital diets (or for that matter any low-calorie crash diet) are said to have "succeeded in overcoming obesity" but follow-up studies show people who manage to lose weight under such programs almost always return to their original status or become even more obese.[289]

What obese persons need is what all persons who lack bountiful energy need: recourse to a predominately carbohydrate diet as a way of life. While research shows carbohydrate-rich diets are usually effective in bringing about weight losses, the nature of the carbohydrate and the degree to which the carbohydrate is processed may affect the degree of success of such diets. The amount of salt and caffeine-containing beverages consumed and the pattern of eating may also be important.[290]

Rats show no signs of becoming obese when their carbohydrate is derived from the starch of whole grains. But when rats are fed refined grains a "fair proportion" of the animals become obese. A fair proportion of *humans* taking refined grains become obese also.[291]

U.S. Department of Agriculture researchers found sugar has a more fattening effect on rats than refined grains. An authority on obesity confirmed the Agriculture Department's findings, but noted fat caused much greater weight increases in rats than sugar. Nevertheless, sugar is implicated in obesity, and replacing sugar with cyclamates in the diets of rats served only to increase the animals' tendency to become obese by boosting food intake.[292]

Sugar has an unpleasant taste for most humans when their blood sugar is elevated (e.g. following a meal). But tests show sugar retains its strong appeal for obese individuals even after prolonged eating. Children taking typical Western diets often exhibit an insatiable desire for sugar, and sugar is believed to play a major role in a rising incidence of obesity among young children.[293]

The very high salt content of typical Western diets result in almost incessant thirst. Animal studies show increased water intake results in increased food intake so the large amount of water required to offset the salt-fest may be partially responsible for the excess of calories in normal diets. Americans usually try to bury their thirst with soft drinks, milk, "regular" coffee, beer and the like which tend to promote obesity directly. Coffee and cola drinks add to the threat of obesity not only through the sugar they contain, but through their high content of caffeine. Caffeine like sugar, tends to depress serum glucose (blood sugar) which boosts the appetite.[294]

A simple way to eliminate the desire for liquid is to switch to a salt-free, whole-foods vegetarian diet. It takes only a brief period to allow the taste buds to acclimate to the lack of salt and after the transition, one is able, usually for the first time, to enjoy the subtle, true tastes of food.[295]

It is alleged that obesity is related to eating too few meals and too much at those meals. However, studies used to back this contention involved force feeding animals (by putting a tube down the animals' throats and pumping food in) once or twice a day so they take as much food as animals fed *ad libitum* i.e., given unlimited free access to food. When animals are "meal fed," that is given all they want to eat but only during two one-hour periods per day, they eat considerably less than animals fed *ad libitum*. The meal feeding program yields some favorable metabolic changes unless their diet is high in fat, but the procedure has been criticized on the basis that it tends to elevate serum lipids. However, the difference between the lipid levels of meal-fed animals and "nibblers" is evidently cyclic, and there is no evidence that meal-feeding tends in any way to promote atherosclerosis. In fact, meal-fed rats have been found to live considerably longer than nibbling ones and the meal eaters tend to weigh less and accumulate less body fat.[296]

The possibility that eating less frequently will bring about lesser food intake for humans seems not to have been considered. A study involving six young women taking two, three or nine meals a day showed no effects in body weight or metabolism but the caloric intake of the subjects was controlled so as to remain equal. An attempt to feed children with gastrointestinal disorders seven to ten times a day had disappointing results, and it should be remembered that it is in the U.S. and Europe, where people nibble constantly, that obesity and cardiovascular disease is a problem.[297]

It is ludicrous to suggest, as some have, that the many obese people who gorge themselves from six p.m. until midnight and then avoid food for 18 hours are eating one meal a day. It would be equally absurd to suggest the slim, strong, long-living Abkhasians should eat more than three times per day. No prescribed pattern of eating is going to eradicate obesity, and from animal studies it appears the many meals a day program is the worst possible pattern to try. Eating once or twice a day seems to enhance the activity levels of humans and it produces greater enjoyment of meals.[298]

HYPOGLYCEMIA

Hypoglycemia (low blood glucose) is a condition which affects the mind and body. It results in a host of emotional disturbances and is the principle symptom of debilitating multiple sclerosis. Paradoxically the condition is both widespread and easy to cure. Hypoglycemia usually arises through an excess of the hormone insulin which tends to depress serum glucose. But a cure requires no injections or surgery, only a little understanding and restraint.[299]

Insulin-induced hypoglycemia is tied to high-sugar intake. Sugar is rapidly absorbed into the bloodstream and initiates a rapid rise in serum glucose which forces a rapid rise in insulin levels. This is followed by a precipitous fall in glucose entering the bloodstream as the last of the sugar is absorbed from the intestines. Since this fall occurs in the presence of high concentrations of insulin, serum glucose levels tend to become very depressed. When sugar intake is increased to the point where sugar serves as the principle source of energy, fasting serum glucose ebbs almost daily and hypoglycemic levels may be reached in a matter of weeks. Lesser sugar intakes work in a similar fashion, albeit slower, and it has been estimated that up to 20% of all Americans suffer from hypoglycemia. The danger of insulin-induced hypoglycemia is increased by cola drinks, coffee, tea and other products containing caffeine. Caffeine is believed to make the pancreas more sensitive, hence excrete greater amounts of insulin. Numerous drugs and even nutritional supplements can lead to temporary rises in serum glucose or disturb insulin output so as to cause hypoglycemia.[300]

Alcohol plays a special role in hypoglycemia. Alcohol is absorbed even more rapidly than sugar, and alcohol serves as fuel for the brain and nervous system as soon as it enters the bloodstream. The brain and nervous system normally use a great deal of glucose, but the presence of alcohol causes a sharp reduction in their glucose uptake. Thus serum glucose tends to rise which brings on a rise in insulin. The situation remains unchanged until the brain and nerves have used up the alcohol in the blood and turn again to glucose for their energy needs. At this point serum insulin is still high so that cells of all types actively grab up glucose from the blood and the result is hypoglycemia. Worst to suffer are the brain and nervous system cells: from being overfed, indeed from being burned up by alcohol, they are suddenly left with an inadequate supply of energy. The result is a strong desire for more alcohol.[301]

Since hypoglycemia affects first and foremost the brain, it results in various mental disturbances. Over 90% of a group of 220 so-called neurotics were found to be suffering from hypoglycemia. Neurotics are characteristically unresponsive to others, turning their attention on themselves and their problems. A brain without an adequate fuel supply is limited in scope and capacity, and treating a hypoglycemic with psychiatry alone is to deal with only a part of the problem.[302]

The first symptoms of hypoglycemia are hunger, weakness and sweating. It may then lead to dizziness, shaking and a severe headache but it is sure to result in reduced mental output. Sometimes the latter results in confusion or incoherent speech, but there is no assurance a hypoglycemic will remain docile. Indeed, he may resort to extreme violence: Hitler took increasing quantities of sugar, alcohol and drugs during the last years of his brutal reign; Lee Harvey Oswald left at his warehouse perch at least one empty coke bottle; and Charles Whitman, the infamous sniper who gunned down a dozen passing Austinites from the tower of the University of Texas, left behind numerous candy wrappers, suggesting both Oswald and Whitman needed boosts in blood glucose.[303]

Rarely are the serum glucose levels of criminals measured, but when the seemingly mild-mannered Anthony Pafa brutally killed the five-year-old child of a neighbor in 1947, his serum glucose was examined and, indeed, he had hypoglycemia. Fortunately there are few hypoglycemics whose disturbances lead to such extremes. Most simply experience chronic fatigue with lack of interest in their work and life in general. When a large group of patients whose principle symptom was fatigue were given tests for impaired carbohydrate metabolism, it was found many had low fasting serum glucose levels; the serum glucose of all patients rose rapidly after an intravenous glucose load but in a matter of three hours, the glucose levels of all patients became depressed. The study not only indicates how often hypoglycemia may be the basis for lethargy but shows the conventional method of detecting hypoglycemia is unreliable.[304]

Anyone who finds life dull, repetitive and meaningless may be suffering from hypoglycemia. Anyone who is "lazy," inactive, slow, distant, aloof, noncommunicative, frequently depressed or just dull may have low blood glucose. Further evidence of low blood sugar is seen in the need for coffee or cola drinks to "get going," the desire for candy, cookies, cakes, pies, ice cream and other sweets for a "lift" or the need for beer, wine or other forms of alcohol to overcome "daily stresses" and to gain "peace of mind." It goes without saying that reliance on powders, pills, vapors, etc., be they prescribed, readily available or illicit, may be a reaction to low blood sugar; as may be anger, aggression and withdrawal.[305]

The cure for hypoglycemia is the elimination of its cause. In most cases the cause is sugar and sweets, but the situation is likely to be aggravated by high intake of refined grains. The latter are absorbed not a great deal less rapidly than sugar, and like sugar, they tend to deprive the body of nutrients necessary for carbohydrate metabolism. A host of vitamins and at least two minerals are involved directly in carbohydrate metabolism and a lack of any of these nutrients leads to decreases in the utilization of glucose. While hypoglycemia is not always involved, the brain and nervous system react to a declining ability to utilize glucose in the same way they react to hypoglycemia: by failing to perfrom their designated roles due to a lack of energy.[306]

Hypoglycemia (low blood sugar) and hyperglycemia (diabetes) are simply two sides of the same coin: both reflect abnormal carbohydrate metabolism. The symptoms differ to the extent diabetes is related to a large number of "physical disorders" such as atherosclerosis, obesity, hypertension, etc., while hypoglycemia is related to a broad spectrum of mental conditions as well as such physical maladies as alcoholism, asthma, ulcers, rheumatic fever and multiple sclerosis. Whole-foods low-fat sugar-free diets have been effective in curing both hyperglycemia and hypoglycemia related disorders. Hypoglycemia itself responds almost overnight to a diet of the SGA type.[307]

EMOTIONAL DISORDERS

One cannot but be impressed by reports of the fun-loving, outgoing Hunzas. These vibrantly healthy, long-living people live at peace with themselves, their own community and outsiders alike. They evidence no feelings of aggression or depression: crime, war and suicide are unknown to them. It is easy to dismiss their joyful mien as "primitive." Indeed they have no hamburger stands nor ice cream parlors, as they almost never eat meat and never eat sugar.

They have no supermarkets or health food shops for they grow their own food and choose a diet with adequate amounts of the necessary nutrients. The Hunzas have no hospitals or doctors and they have no need for lawyers, police or judges since they have no disputes. The Hunzas have no lifts to carry them up the mighty Himalayas, but they seem to enjoy the climbing tremendously, making a virtual dance of the ascent. They have no automobiles or jumbo jets to take them away from the environment they love. Not all "civilized" observers can appreciate the richness of the lives of such people; fewer yet regard such life-styles as reasonable alternatives to their own. But the inner peace of the Hunzas is an oasis of emotional stability in a world of chaos, fear, anxiety, aggression and despair.[308]

Half of those going to doctors in the United States are thought to be victims of a troubled mind. "Stress" is often blamed for the nation's anxieties and indeed the stresses induced by dietary excesses and deficiencies can affect the mind. During an extended tour of societies living in simple ways, Dr. W. A. Price watched an isolated group of islanders lose their joyful, outgoing manner when for the first time they were exposed to sugar and refined flour. With the introduction of the Western staples the islanders went from a state of radiant happiness to morbid depression which in time led to broken homes and suicide. Then, after two years, it had become unprofitable to trade with the islands so the sugar and flour-bearing ships ceased to come, and the natives returned to their previous ways: individuals once more radiated happiness, marital problems vanished and suicides ceased. Only a host of rotted teeth was left as a reminder of the days of sugar and white bread.[309]

Eliminating sugar, cutting way down on refined flour and doing without caffeine-containing drinks (coffee, tea, colas, etc.) has led to some amazing changes in Americans also. Dr. E. M. Abrahamson reported (1) A 48 year-old woman who had become "morose and then greatly depressed" recovered from her despondency and became energetic and gay when she was taken off of sugar and coffee. (2) A man of the same age who brooded until he attempted suicide whereupon he was placed on the sugarless, caffeine-free diet; in less than three weeks he felt "entirely fit" and he continued to improve. (3) A 69 year-old hypochondriac woman who made the rounds of allergists until she met a doctor who had her drop sugar from her diet which not only eliminated her (real) allergetic state but ended her hypochondria. (4) A survivor of the infamous Bataan death march who had digestive problems and frequent nightmares in which he re-experienced his prison camp beatings until he stopped using sugar and caffeine. With the change he "became vigorous in both mind and body." (5) Others who had such symptoms as nervousness, fatigue and irritability, claustrophobia, "preoccupation with a general demise," etc. and who brought their problems to an end by dropping sugar and caffeine from their diets.[310]

Sugar and caffeine are not the only "mind blowers," however. Dr. G. Watson, author of *Nutrition and Your Mind*, found a girl suffering from schizophrenia and periodic catatonia experienced rapid reversal of her conditions with a low-fat, low-protein diet even though she continued to eat sugar. Watson noted a high-fat, high-protein diet reversed the condition of a girl who had undergone shock treatments for a psychotic condition; predictably, though the growth-stimulating diet led in time to new emotional disturbances. In addition to changes in fat, carbohydrate and protein, Watson used niacin, pantothenic acid and other supplements to treat patients.[311]

Impaired carbohydrate metabolism should be regarded as a prime suspect in almost any mental or emotional disorder. Anything leading to a reduction in the supply of utilizable carbohydrate (as glucose) for the always hungry brain and nerves can lead to problems. Unlike other body cells, the cells of the brain and nervous system cannot burn fat so they must rely almost exclusively on glucose for energy. In the absence of glucose most cells, especially those of muscle tissue, are relatively impermeable to glucose but brain and nerve cells are prepared to take up glucose at all times. The rate at which the cells of the brain and nervous system take up glucose depends on the level of glucose in the blood, and a low level of blood glucose (hypoglycemia) can lead to rapid damage to the brain and nerves which results in all manner of emotional disturbances.[312]

The ability of the brain to function properly depends on its capacity to utilize glucose as well as there being an adequate level of serum glucose. The ability to utilize glucose depends on adequate supplies of numerous vitamins and minerals. Inadequate levels of any one of at least seven nutrients (niacin, thiamin, biotin, pantothenic acid, riboflavin, magnesium and manganese) known to be involved in carbohydrate metabolism leads to mental disturbances. Whether or not hypoglycemia accompanies these disturbances is unclear. What is clear, and disturbing, is the following:[313]

1. The normal U.S. diet is dangerously low in at least four of these nutrients, namely biotin, pantothenic acid, manganese and magnesium.

2. The emotional and neurological disturbances brought about by deficiences of these four nutrients include behavior and states of mind so common that they have come to be accepted as normal (e.g. restlessness, boredom, lassitude, depression, irritability, insomnia and somnolence).

3. Many North Americans and Europeans may also be taking inadequate amounts of niacin, thiamin and riboflavin. Unfortunately, the cause of emotional disturbances resulting from a lack of one of these vitamins may fail to be recognized because of a lack of physical symptoms.

4. Prolonged deficiency of any nutrient upon which both carbohydrate metabolism and emotional stability depend can lead to such extremes as overt madness, widespread nerve degeneration or extensive brain damage.

5. The U.S. diet is also very low in chromium which is necessary for proper carbohydrate metabolism but for which deficiency symptoms have not been established.

6. The U.S. diet is exceedingly low in a number of other nutrients which are not involved directly in carbohydrate metabolism, but which are necessary for emotional stability. Included are vitamin A, vitamin C, pyridoxine, vitamin E and folacin, and deficiency symptoms range from confusion and severe depression to nerve degeneration and brain damage.[314]

In Appendix 4 it is shown that normal diets are staggeringly low in biotin, pantothenic acid, manganese and magnesium. The lack of dietary biotin might be offset by synthesis of the vitamin by intestinal bacteria but excesses of sugar, fat and drugs (especially prescribed ones) in normal diets render intestinal synthesis a highly unreliable source. The easiest way to boost pantothenic acid intake is to boost vegetable intake. The only rich food sources of manganese or magnesium are whole grains, soybeans, legumes, green leaf vegetables and nuts.[315]

Niacin deficiency leads to loss of memory, hallucinations, persecution complexes and severe depression. Niacin supplements have been effective in treating various emotional disorders thereby indicating a deficiency in spite of the fact refined grains are fortified with niacin. Refined grain products are also fortified with thiamin, but mental depression and confusion are sometimes alleviated by thiamin administration also. Thiamin has also been used in treating neuritis, neuralgia and other diseases of the central nervous system. As we know normal diets are proposterously high in fat, and the combination of high fat and low riboflavin may lead to degenerative changes in the myelin sheaths of fibers in the nerves. Sprouts and greens are exceedingly rich in niacin, thiamin and riboflavin, and the SGA diet contains a high multiple of needs for all three vitamins.[316]

Chromium is found primarily in whole grains, legumes and other seeds. Intake of grain products has been slipping for over 50 years, and the grain products that are ingested are almost always refined which tends to rid them of chromium.[317]

Although vitamin E plays no known role in carbohydrate metabolism, vitamin E deficiency is associated with diseases of the central nervous system, brain damage, degeneration of the spinal cord and paralysis in animals. Normal diets are very low in vitamin E and an excess of fat tends to worsen the nerve degeneration seen in rats deprived of the vitamin. Sprouted soybeans, sprouted wheat and greens are excellent sources of vitamin E.[318]

Peripheral neurological damage has been related to lack of folacin, and folacin deficient patients experience an emotional lift upon receiving the vitamin. Low folacin levels in the blood is strong evidence of folacin deficiency, and three separate studies of psychiatric cases showed more than half the patients had low levels of serum folacin. Most vegetarian diets are high in folacin: greens and bean sprouts are the richest sources.[319]

Pyridoxine deficiency was seen to result in mental confusion, and pyridoxine has been used to treat poliomyelitis, multiple sclerosis and other nerve related disorders.[320]

Mineral imbalances and deficiencies seemingly unrelated to carbohydrate metabolism can cause neurological changes also. The transmission of nerve impulses depends on the balance of sodium and potassium in fluids within and surrounding cells. Excess salt intake may set the stage for sodium depletion which has been observed in patients with certain diseases of the central nervous system and brain disorders. Copper is required for the synthesis of the myelin sheath surrounding nerve fibers. Copper deficient animals showed losses of myelin in brain and motor tracts of the spinal cord. They also exhibit a lack of appetite and a swayback condition similar to multiple sclerosis in man.[321]

The path to protection against nutritionally induced emotional disorders is clear. It involves abstinence from sugar, a low-fat intake and healthy amounts of the required vitamins and minerals, especially those involved in carbohydrate metabolism. Greens and sprouts have outstanding levels of all the minerals and vitamins associated with emotional stability. The combination of sprouts, greens and seaweed, the SGA diet, contains almost no sucrose (sugar) and a very safe level of fat.[322]

MULTIPLE SCLEROSIS

Degeneration of the myelin sheaths surrounding nerves and hypoglycemia are the hallmarks of a disease known as multiple sclerosis. In a process that lasts years, multiple sclerosis begins with abnormal neurological signs then progresses to a period during which physical capacity begins to wane and finally to a stage of complete physical disability and death.[323]

Multiple sclerosis was first seen in France in the latter part of the 19th century. It was first reported in the United States in 1898 and now ranks as the most common disease of the central nervous system among Americans 20 to 50 years of age. The disease affects an estimated quarter million persons in the United States, and the number is rising rapidly. If nerve degeneration reaches the proportions of degeneration of the arteries there will no longer be a question of which adults have the disease, only questions of what stage it is in.[324]

Like most degenerative diseases multiple sclerosis is most prevalent in the U.S. and Western Europe. It is uncommon in Eastern Europe, the USSR, Arab countries, China, North Korea and Islands in the Pacific. One of the most revealing aspects of its occurrence is its rarity among African Negroes and high incidence among U.S. Blacks. The rate for U.S. blacks matches that of Caucasians in North America.[325]

Deficiencies of any of a number of vitamins and minerals including vitamins A, C and E, thiamin, biotin, pantothenic acid, magnesium, manganese, copper and pyridoxine can lead to destruction of the myelin sheath of nerves. It was noted previously that a high fat intake combined with low levels of riboflavin can also lead to sheath destruction. Saturated fats may be still another dietary item leading to sheath degeneration and hypoglycemia may set the stage for sheath destruction by leaving nerve cells short of an energy source. The presence of hypoglycemia in multiple sclerosis suggests a high sugar intake plus a host of mineral and vitamin deficiencies may be involved in the etiology of the disease. There is the strongest kind of evidence that a high fat intake is also involved.[326]

The medical profession regards multiple sclerosis as incurable but modifications in the diet have been successful in arresting the disease and several B-vitamins have been found to be useful in treating the disease. Best results seem to have come from the Waerland lacto-vegetarian diet and the Evers diet which begins as a vegetarian diet but later admits small quantities of raw pork.[327]

Orotic acid (vitamin B_{13}) which is found in root vegetables, especially beets, has been used to treat multiple sclerosis in Europe but reports are vague about the effectiveness of the treatment. Supplemental pyridoxine (vitamin B_6) reportedly resulted in "some success" with multiple sclerosis, and Vitamin B_6 deficiency has been implicated directly in hypoglycemia and nervous disorders. In relating multiple sclerosis to B_6 deficiency, two researchers noted environmental pollution by carbon monoxide from automobiles tends to increase the requirements for B_6. In any case there is every indication the B_6 level of the normal diet is quite low (*see Pyridoxine section in Appendix 4*). On the other hand, the levels of a number of nutrients which may be necessary to prevent multiple sclerosis, including vitamin E, biotin, pantothenic acid, magnesium and manganese appear to be critically low in normal diets (*see appropriate section in Appendix 4*). While the addition of B_6 and orotic acid to a standard diet may be helpful, broader nutritional approaches to multiple sclerosis have a sounder theoretical basis, and they have yielded more impressive results.[328]

Dr. E. M. Abrahamson had a number of multiple sclerosis patients eliminate sugar, pastries, candy, cake, ice cream and other items to which sugar is added. He also had them cut out coffee, tea, "cola" beverages, beer, wine, most hard liquors and selected fruits. Response to Abrahamson's diet is said to be varied but Abrahamson reported 12 patients showed little sign of multiple sclerosis upon adopting his dietary changes.[329]

Dr. R. L. Swank of the University of Oregon Medical School, treated 146 multiple sclerosis patients with a low-fat diet for a number of years. The diet contained 30 to 40 grams of fat with as little as 50 grams of protein and a single vitamin capsule containing several of the B-vitamins plus vitamins A, C and D. If treated in the first two to three years of the disease, before severe disability had developed, response was excellent. Almost 90% of those who began the low-fat diets during the early stages of the disease improved over the succeeding years and a high percentage avoided deterioration for the 20 years he monitored their progress. Over two thirds of those for whom the disease had reached an intermediate stage avoided deterioration after an average of more than seven years on the diet, but only a third of those who had allowed the disease to reach the state of severe disability did not continue to decline. On the whole, there were marked reductions in the death rate and the frequency and severity of aggravation. And those who took the lowest amounts of animal fats apparently responded better than those who took their fat as lard, butter, etc.[330]

According to one group of researchers, diets high in animal protein tend to promote multiple sclerosis and experiments by others showed multiple sclerosis patients tended to improve significantly when animal fat was replaced by corn and soy oil in their diets and their intake of several B-vitamins was increased.[331]

Dr. E. Evers has treated over 15,000 multiple sclerosis sufferers with a diet consisting of a small amount of sprouted grain, whole wheat bread, raw oat flakes, fruit, uncooked roots, raw milk, butter and honey, and in some cases, raw eggs. Nicotine, coffee, tea, cocoa, sugar, salt, condiments and confectionaries are strictly forbidden. According to the editors of Journal of the American Medical Association (JAMA) "The (Evers) diet has not been tested utilizing a modern statistical design," but Evers claims multiple sclerosis is 100% curable for persons who come to him within five years of the onset of the disease. However, Dr. E. Waerland claims progress is slow and sometimes fails under the Evers regime. She notes Evers gives certain patients raw meat and raw eggs and excludes potatoes and green leaves from his "otherwise fine diet." Waerland has her own diet for multiple sclerosis patients, and it is said to attain quick results but it does not include sprouts, as the Evers diet does, nor does it *specify* the use of leaf vegetables. It may be weakened further by the inclusion of some oil, dairy products and cooked grains.[332]

There is a sound theoretical basis and strong experimental evidence that multiple sclerosis is a disease resulting from diets containing excesses of animal products, fat and sugar and having low levels of certain vitamins and minerals. These findings have ample epidemological support.[333]

Swank noted per capita fat intake ranged from 105 to 151 grams per day in nine nations with a high prevalence of multiple sclerosis; per capita fat intake was only 24 to 60 grams per day in nine countries with a low prevalence of the disease. But sugar intake is highly correlated with fat intake so the prevalence of multiple sclerosis should closely parallel sugar consumption also.[334]

It seems quite clear that a diet offering strong supplies of the vitamins and minerals associated with the integrity of the nervous system, especially those which prevent the degeneration of the myelin sheaths of nerves, is vital to the prevention and cure of multiple sclerosis. But the diet should contain no sugar, sweetened foods, alcohol, stimulants or refined foods and it should be very low in total fat with a minimum fraction of total fat from animal sources. A diet based on sprouts, greens and a little seaweed (*SGA diet*) offers rich amounts of every nutrient known to be involved in any aspect of the nervous system and carbohydrate metabolism. This includes not only vitamins A, C and the members of the B complex, which Swank used, but vitamin E, magnesium, manganese and copper. An SGA-type diet offers much more in the form of high levels of promising new B-vitamins (like B_{13}) and abundant amounts of all vitamins and minerals believed to be essential in human nutrition. The SGA diet is lower in total fat than the Swank or Evers diets, contains no animal fat, and unlike the Waerland diet, is completely free of sugar. It is also free of alcohol, stimulants and refined foods. Thus, it represents substantial improvements over the most successful treatments for multiple sclerosis and it is highly unlikely anyone taking such a food mix could ever develop "incurable" multiple sclerosis.[335]

CYSTIC FIBROSIS

Disturbed carbohydrate metabolism is said to be the primary cause of cystic fibrosis which afflicts an estimated one in 600 children at birth. All who contract cystic fibrosis develop the disease at birth or in the first few years of life and few of those afflicted reach adulthood.[336]

Children with cystic fibrosis tend to have voracious appetites, but they are unable to gain weight. Presumably this condition is related to failure of cells to utilize carbohydrates since the pancreas is often, if not always, impaired. Cystic fibrosis invariably involves losses of protein and fats in conjunction with severe evacuation problems. The breathing apparatus is also almost always impaired. Children with cystic fibrosis tend to develop persistant coughs that fail to rid the respiratory tract of a sticky mucus formation. There is evidence the condition is related to impaired carbohydratic metabolism by the cells of the lungs.[337]

Since cystic fibrosis is related to impaired carbohydrate metabolism, pancreatic insufficiency and possibly excretory and digestive disorders, it would be expected that a low-fat diet with an abundant supply of necessary vitamins and minerals would be effective in treating the disease. If such a diet were taken as whole foods it should offer relief to the pancreas. Pancreatic supplements were effective in arresting degeneration in 20 patients, and autopsies have identified specific deficiencies of vitamins A and E as well as folacin and vitamin B_{12} in cystic fibrosis patients. It was found that both low-fat diets and supplements of vitamins A and C brought about improvements in the condition of patients. Recently the parents of what was diagnosed as a "serious case" of cystic fibrosis in Texas decided to reject the recommendations of antibiotic-pushers and to rely on "natural foods and vitamin supplements." So successful was the treatment that the local chapter of the National Cystic Fibrosis Foundation gave a grant to a major university to study the relationship between diet and cystic fibrosis.[338]

What is clearly needed to wipe out cystic fibrosis is an overhaul of the diets of prospective parents. The disease was not recognized until 1938, and its response to even modest dietary changes is strong evidence the disease is a carry over from excesses and deficiencies in the mother's diet. Until major adjustments are made, however, we are still going to face cystic fibrosis. For infants beyond age six months or so a combination of raw, dark green leafy vegetables and raw sprouts just might cure the disease. The mix is loaded with vitamin A, C, E and folacin, and it is low in fat. It contains exceedingly rich amounts of all of the vitamins and minerals required for carbohydrate metabolism, and it has an adequate supply of good quality proteins. Hopefully parents who first use the SGA mix to treat cystic fibrosis will treat themselves, as well as their children.[339]

4 / aging

LONGEVITY

The primary reason scientists are paying so much attention to the Vilcabambans, Hunzas and Abkhasians is that their life spans are far greater than those of Americans and Europeans. Theories to explain their longevity abound but a striking similarity in the diets of the three groups seems to be a little hard for meat-eating theorists to digest. All three groups border on vegetarianism. The Abkhasians take flesh only once or twice a week, the Vilcabambas take even less animal protein than the Abkhasians and the Hunzas normally take meat only once a year. The Abkhasians regularly consume a low-fat fermented milk product, not unlike buttermilk, but the Hunzas take almost no animal products whatsoever. Elderly Vilcabambans were found to be taking only 35 to 38 grams of protein per day and their fat intake was a scant 12 to 19 grams per day. All three groups take at least a third fewer calories than North Americans and Europeans of comparable ages.[340]

The Hunzas, Abkhasians and Vilcabambas not only live much longer than inhabitants of "advanced" societies, but they enjoy full, active lives throughout their many years. They work and play at 80 and beyond; most of those who reach their 100th birthday continue to be active and retirement is unheard of. The absence of growth promoters in their diets engenders slower growth and slim, compact body frames. With age, wisdom accumulates but physical degeneration is limited so the senior citizens of these remote societies have something unique to contribute to the lives of others. They are revered.[341]

The experience of the Seventh Day Adventists in the U.S. makes it difficult to dismiss the superior health and longer life spans of remote groups as being the consequences of "genetic differences" or "lack of stress." The Adventists are inclined to vegetarianism and evidence far less susceptibility to degenerative disease than their fellow countrymen. The average life span of the Adventists is much greater than non-Adventists living in the same (stress-ridden) areas. If the Adventists are genetically superior they must have derived that status from their ways of eating and living for they come of the same hetero-geneous stock as other North Americans. And if "stress" is taken to mean something in their surroundings, the Adventists must be as-sumed to get their share. In any case stress does not seem to shorten life spans: the presidents of the United States's biggest corporations have far lower than average mortality rates and in Norway stress re-sulting from deprivation and subjugation by German occupation forces during WW II was accompanied by lower death rates. On the other hand the Norwegians ate lesser amounts of animal products and refined foods during the period.[342]

These findings raise the question of why all groups who eat less and take little animal food do not outlive Westerners. Presumably the answer lies in the nutritional completeness of the diets of the Abkhasians, Hunzas, Vilcabambans and those Seventh Day Ad-ventists who follow vegetarian diets. A close look at the diets of these groups shows they get much higher than normal supplies of the necessary vitamins and minerals. They take no sugar, refined cereal grains, canned foods or factory made items and they abstain from drugs, including coffee. The Abkhasians take a small amount of a low alcohol, local wine but it can hardly be a contributor to their good health, as some have suggested. Salt intake is kept at a mini-mum by these people and they do not, as a rule, eat between meals.[343]

Striking increases in longevity and curtailment of "aging" are to be expected from low-calorie, low-fat, modest-protein diets which are not deficient in vitamins and minerals. Some 50 years of research have been devoted to feeding vast numbers of animals restricted amounts of food, low levels of fat and protein, etc. and the results are always the same: cutting intake leads to marked increases in life span and the longer life span is accompanied by dramatic reductions in degenerative disease and a vibrant, active bearing.[344]

There is no obesity among the Abkhasians, Hunzas or Vilcabam-bans and reduced weight means added life span and added weight means shortened life expectancy in both humans and animals. A 30% reduction in weight raises life expectancy an estimated 40%. Cutting the food intake of animals even at advanced ages brings tremendous increases in life span. And reducing intake of factors which promote obesity, particularly fat, protein and refined foods tends to increase life span even when calories are not restricted.[345]

High fat intake has been shown to reduce the life spans of laboratory animals while raising carbohydrate intake was shown to increase their life spans. Lowering protein intake tends to increase the life span of rats while their life span was cut substantially when sugar was added to their diets. "Meal feeding" tends to cause a voluntary reduction of food intake, and the life span of rats allowed to eat *ad libitum* was 17% less than those fed a single two-hour "meal" each day. When high fat and sugar were both introduced into the diets of rabbits, their life span was cut by almost 50%.[346]

The life expectancy of animals is also reduced by failure to provide optimal amounts of vitamins and minerals. Levels simply adequate to avoid deficiency symptoms may not be adequate to promote long life. An increase over apparently adequate levels in a single B-vitamin led to an 18% increase in life span of rats. By taking a diet of whole grains, vegetables, milk and fruit, the Abkhasians get at least adequate levels of all the vitamins and minerals known to be needed. Americans clearly do not (*see Appendix 4 for details*). Happily, it is possible to go further than the Abkhasians or the Hunzas or the Vilcabambas in choosing vitamin-and mineral-rich foods. By replacing cooked whole grains with raw bean and grain sprouts, most vitamin levels are boosted threefold or more and minerals become more utilizable. Raising intake of greens elevates intake of almost all of the necessary vitamins and minerals and including seaweed in the diet eliminates the need for any animal food while adding to the diet a host of micronutrients. A good diet promotes a long life unmarked by the throes of so-called "aging."[347]

AGING

Aging is usually taken to mean a collection of chronic conditions which most North Americans and Europeans develop and whose symptoms normally do not appear until late in life. Conditions associated with "aging" include immobility, loss of strength, stooped posture, inflammation and inflexibility of joints, impairment of sight and hearing, roughening of skin, loss of mental capacities and numerous internal disorders including hardening of the arteries, impaired digestion and stone formations. One by one these "aspects of aging" are being scrutinized and related to something more controllable than years—something called diet.[348]

Diet should have become suspect in aging when it was first recognized that aging is a process in which calcium is shifted from the bones to the soft tissues of the body. Wrinkling of the skin is a visible sign of calcium build-ups in soft tissue; cataracts represent calcium deposits in the lens of the eyes; arthritis is related to the transfer of bone calcium to joints; kidney, urinary and bladder stones are often made up of calcium-based deposits; and advanced atherosclerosis or "hardening of the arteries" involves the deposition of calcium and other minerals into fatty deposits along the interior walls of the arteries. It is surprising that so much research has been devoted to the sources of lipids in atherosclerosis while so little attention seems to be given the minerals involved, particularly calcium, which is credited with the sclerosis, or hardening, itself.[349]

OSTEOPOROSIS

The calcium in atherosclerotic deposits and indeed the calcium in all soft tissue deposits is derived from calcium in the bloodstream which is elevated by loss of calcium from the bones. Loss of bone calcium or rarification is the essence of osteoporosis, which is one of the principle diseases of aging. With the loss of calcium (osteoporosis) bones are left springy, fragile and weak. This results in back pain and frequent fractures, particularly of the hip; eventually it causes a loss of height and stooping as the weakened vertebrae yield to the body load.[350]

A study at the University of Tennessee indicates that osteoporosis begins in women following menopause whereas in men it may not occur until age 60 or later. Other studies indicate bone decalcification may commence much earlier in both sexes. Be that as it may, the disease seems to eventually afflict and debilitate a major segment of those taking meat-based diets, and two eminent physicians vowed the "association (of meat-based diets) with the increasing incidence of bone-mass loss with age is inescapable." Working under the sponsorship of the U.S. Public Health Service and Harvard University, Drs. Ammon Wachman and Daniel Bernstein went on to say that "it

might be worth while to consider" a diet emphasizing fruits, vegetables and moderate amounts of milk.[351]

Osteoporosis occurs earlier and tends to be more pronounced in
women, and British investigators found the average bone density of a
group of lacto-vegetarian women was greater than that of meat-eating women of the same age. The essentially lacto-vegetarian Abkhasians give no evidence of losing their bone integrity with age. Dr.
Sula Benet noted Abkhasians 80 to 119 years of age remain active and
work with erect postures while enjoying walking and swimming for
added exercise. The men are described as slim, but not frail, and their
enjoyment of horseback riding yields enough broken bones to show
healing is rapid and complete. Not only do the Abkhasians maintain
their bone structure, but they seem to be bothered little by calcium
deposits in their soft tissues; the aged have wrinkled skin, but they
rarely develop atherosclerotic heart disease, and there are no reports
of kidney and bladder stones, arthritis or cataracts.[352]

A study of South African Bantu men and women in their seventies
showed that they had a lesser incidence of hip fracture and severe collapse of the vertebrae than South African whites taking conventional
Western diets. A study of elderly persons in Surinam (South America) revealed they rarely experienced spontaneous fracture of the vertebrae, while over 25% of a group of 136 elderly Philadelphians were
found to suffer from the malady. Less than a third of the Surinams
had distinct osteoporosis; presumably osteoporosis afflicted just
about all of the aged Philadelphians.[353]

Evidently sparse diets like those of the Bantu and Surinams induce
lesser amounts of bone demineralization than normal Western diets,
and the essentially vegetarian diets of the Hunzas and Abkhasians
seem to afford them complete freedom from bone rarification. There
is mounting evidence that meat, eggs, fish and other "protein foods"
are the principle causes of osteoporosis in the West.[354]

Most foods which are high in protein are also high in minerals that
tend to acidify the blood. Meat, eggs and fish are especially rich in
the acid-forming minerals so if animal products are not accompanied
by substantial amounts of fruit and vegetables to counter the acidity,
the bones are forced to give up calcium as a buffering agent. Without
some means of keeping the blood essentially neutral, individuals
would die. Exhibit L1 gives the acid-forming capacity of some com-

Food Reform

mon food items while Exhibit L2 gives the base-forming capacity of
a number of vegetables, legumes, fruits and nuts. It is obvious
normal Western diets tend to be acidic while vegetable-based diets
are alkaline in nature.[355]

Exhibit L1

Acid Forming Capacities of Selected Foods

FOOD	ACIDITY M-EQUIV. PER 100g
Meat	
Beef, sirloin, roast, lean only	23.5
Beef steak, grilled	23.5
Ham, boiled, lean only	22.3
Calves' liver, fried	46.9
Bacon, streaky, fried	17.0
Ham, boiled	16.2
Veal, roast	28.5
Chicken, roast	25.4
Seafood	
Haddock, fried	14.0
Sardines, canned	26.5
Oysters, raw	12.4
Eggs, poached	19.7
Cheese, cheddar	5.4
Grains	
Whole wheat, as Shredded Wheat	5.7
Oatmeal porridge	1.5

Source: McCance, R. A. and Widdowson, E. M. "The Composition
of Foods," pp. 22–124, Her Majesty's Stationary Office, 1960.

Exhibit L2

Base Forming Capacities of Selected Foods

FOOD	BASE CAPACITY M-EQUIV. PER 100g
Vegetable	
Spinach, boiled	39.6
Potatoes, baked in skins	10.0
Carrots, raw	9.0
Broccoli, boiled	4.3
Leeks, boiled	5.5
Turnip top, boiled	2.3
Watercress, raw	7.5
Tomatoes, raw	5.6
Legumes*	
Butter beans, raw	35.5
Butter beans, boiled	6.0
Haricot beans, raw	25.5
Haricot beans, boiled	5.0
Broad beans, boiled	1.7
Peas, fresh, raw	1.2
Peas, dried, boiled**	1.2
Fruit	
Apples	3.0
Bananas	7.9
Oranges	6.1
Grapes, white	6.0
Pears, raw	3.4
Raisins, dried	27.0
Figs, dried	36.1
Nuts***	
Almonds	18.3
Brazil Nuts	4.5
Chestnuts	11.3

*Peanuts are acidic
**Canned peas are acidic
***Walnuts are acidic

Source: See Exhibit L1

The relationship between bone demineralization and acid-forming phosphorus in which meat, especially liver, is rich is the focus of increasing concern. Excessive phosphorus intake and low Ca:P ratios both tend to stimulate the parathyroid gland to secrete a hormone which stimulates bone resorption (the passage of bone minerals into the blood). Osteoporosis patients were found to have abnormal parathyroids, and the first stages of osteoporosis are suggestive of a low Ca:P ratio.[356]

Extensive studies with animals have shown that when the level of dietary phosphorus is not excessive, a high Ca:P ratio in the diet will promote strong and lasting bones. When, on the other hand, dietary phosphorus levels are very high bone degeneration is accelerated and the losses can not be counteracted by raising calcium intake because absorption drops sharply as intake is elevated. It is heartening that lowering the phosphorus intake late in life of animals greatly reduces the degree to which bone calcium is lost.[357]

Young women experienced strong calcium retention when taking 1500 milligrams calcium and 800 milligrams of phosphorus per day, but when their phosphorus intake was raised to 1400 milligrams their net calcium retention began to decline and after four weeks their bones were losing calcium. The bone loss of a group of elderly women was ended for 11 months by giving them a supplement of calcium without phosphorus. It is doubtful, though, that calcium supplements would aid milk drinkers or others taking substantial amounts of calcium for large doses of calcium are poorly absorbed.[358]

It seems clear that a diet with a strong Ca:P ratio which is not excessively high in phosphorus should contribute to strong and lasting bones. Bone development usually evokes an image of (cow's) milk but there are better sources of calcium than milk. Part 1 of Exhibit L3 lists a number of whole foods which are higher in calcium and lower in phosphorus than cow's milk. All have a Ca:P ratio more than double that of cow's milk. All are leaf vegetables which are low in calcium-binding oxylates so that the calcium present is readily available. Part 2 of the Exhibit L3 lists some additional rich sources of calcium which, for some reason, fail to qualify for listing in Part 1. Sesame seeds, kelp, cheddar cheese and blackstrap molasses are shown to be very concentrated calcium sources. Part 3 gives the calcium and phosphorus contents and the Ca:P ratios of some common U.S. foodstuffs. The Ca:P ratio of most items, especially meats, is very low. Lettuce is the only item in normal diets with a Ca:P ratio above that of cow's milk but the total calcium content of lettuce is rather low. One expert says the proper Ca:P ratio for the diet as a whole is 1.5:1. The Ca:P ratio of the U.S. diet is about 0.35:1 or less than a quarter of the recommended ratio.[359]

Exhibit L3   Calcium and Phosphorus Content of Selected Foods

Part 1: Whole foods with higher calcium content and lower phosphorus content than cow's milk

FOOD	CALCIUM CONTENT (mg/100g)	PHOSPHORUS CONTENT (mg/100g)	CA:P RATIO
Mustard spinach	210	28	7.5
Turnip greens	246	58	4.2
Amaranth	267	67	4.0
Mustard greens	183	50	3.7
Parsley	203	63	3.2
Collard greens	250	82	3.0
Watercress	151	54	2.8
Cow's Milk	118	93	1.1

Part 2: Additional food products which are good sources of calcium

PRODUCT	CALCIUM (mg/100g)	PHOSPHORUS (mg/100g)	CA:P RATIO
Orange Peels	134	12	11.2
Blackstrap Molasses	684	84	8.2
Kelp	1093	240	4.6
Purslane Leaves	103	39	2.6
Sesame Seeds	1160	616	1.9
Rutabagas	66	39	1.7
Cheddar Cheese	750	478	1.6
Dock	66	41	1.6
Broccoli	103	78	1.3

Part 3: Commonly eaten products.

PRODUCT	CALCIUM (mg/100g)	PHOSPHORUS (mg/100g)	CA:P RATIO
Chicken	10	200	.05
Beef	8	124	.06
Pork	5	88	.06
Haddock	23	197	.12
Liver (calf)	8	333	.02
Enriched white bread	70	87	.81
Poundcake	21	79	.26
Saltines	21	90	.23
Doughnuts	40	190	.21
Tomatoes	13	27	.48
Lettuce	35	26	1.4
French fries	7	67	.10
Apples	7	10	.7
Bananas	8	26	.3

Source: USDA Handbook #8, 1963

High protein intake may be more detrimental to bone calcium than high phosphorus levels. It was reported that rats fed high levels of protein suffered from "calcium depletion" which resulted in a significant reduction in growth. No such effects were seen when the diet was high in carbohydrate. Rats on a meat diet grew but their bones failed to mineralize and rapidly became fragile and rarefied. Resorption of the bone began slowly, then accelerated until the rate of resorption was more than double the rate of bone growth. Protein alone yields an "acid-ash" (i.e. tends to make the blood acidic) and meat is high in both proteins and acid forming phosphorus. At the same time, meat is very low in calcium and meat protein may hinder calcium absorption for it was found liver protein allowed only half as much calcium to enter the bloodstream as did peanut protein.[360]

The results of recent studies at the University of Wisconsin on the effects of high protein on bone resorption in humans deserve careful consideration by advocates of high-protein diets. The studies began when Dr. Nancy Johnson and her colleagues fed six young men a very high 1400 milligrams of calcium per day with a highly favorable 1:1 calcium-phosphorus ratio. When taking 48 grams of protein for 45 days, the young men were evidently in calcium balance. But when their protein intake was boosted to 141 grams per day for 45 days the subjects had a net loss of 84 milligrams of calcium per day not counting sweat losses. Dr. Ruth Walker had almost exactly the same results when she fed nine young men 800 milligrams of calcium and 1000 milligrams of phosphorus per day. On protein levels of 47, 95 and 142 grams per day apparent calcium retention was plus 12, plus 1 and minus 85 milligrams, respectively. There is little doubt that even when taking 95 grams of protein a day the subjects were slowly losing body calcium when sweat losses are included. Even without sweat losses, bone losses with the high protein intake were at a rate which would have resulted in a loss of 3% of total body calcium in a year's time. Dr. Walker noted that Americans had available, on the average, over 100 grams of protein per day.[361]

Recognizing that the Johnson and Walker studies were conducted with relatively high quantities of calcium in the diet, Drs. Chander Anand and Hellen Linkswiler put a group of young men on diets containing 500 milligrams of calcium per day and measured calcium retention with protein again at 47, 95 and 142 grams per day. The subjects retained an average of 131 milligrams of calcium per day on a protein intake of 47 grams per day, but when protein intake was boosted to 95 grams per day they lost an average of 58 milligrams of calcium per day which amounts to about 2% of total body calcium per year. All of the subjects were in negative calcium balance with protein intakes of both 95 grams per day and 142 grams per day (which led to calcium losses averaging 120 milligrams per day).[362]

While a calcium intake of 500 milligrams per day is somewhat lower than that of adults who take liberal amounts of dairy products, the Anand-Linkswiler subjects were taking a very modest 800 milligrams of phosphorus per day which would tend to reduce their susceptibility to bone decomposition. Thus the rather large losses of bone with a protein intake of 95 grams per day suggests many Americans, Britons and Continental Europeans may be experiencing bone degeneration far earlier than realized.[363]

The Anand-Linkswiler study, like those that preceded it, was conducted with diets containing only a third as much meat as North Americans normally take. Thus the acidity of the diets used in these studies may have been considerably below that of normal regimes. Nevertheless the addition of fruits and vegetables to the diet containing 142 grams of protein resulted in a reduction of calcium losses from 120 milligrams per day to 88 milligrams per day. Going to the other extreme, that is putting a group of young men on high meat diets, led to rapid and continuing bone losses.[364]

It was reported that based on international patterns there appears to be an inverse relationship between bone density and the amount of calcium provided in the diet. This reflects the fact that high calcium in the diet on a national scale usually means high intake of dairy products which almost always means high meat intake, and diets high in meat are inherently high in phosphorus and protein with unfavorably low Ca:P ratios.[365]

Inactivity is another, possibly important, factor which may contribute to calcium losses. Exercise tends to markedly reduce urinary calcium losses and increase calcium retention while inactivity tends to cause big increases in urinary calcium losses. However, the process is one that takes time for when five "healthy" young men underwent continuous bed rest for 24 to 30 weeks, they suffered no calcium losses during the first 12 weeks. When they did begin to lose calcium, however, and the rate of their losses eventually became so great that they stood to lose 1% of their total body calcium every two months. Not surprisingly, their losses increased even more when they were given phosphorus supplements. It thus appears that osteoporosis may be accelerated by its very tendency to debilitate. The relationship between inactivity and bone resorption has given rise to the term "inactivity osteoporosis." Children and aging individuals are especially vulnerable to skeleton damage from inactivity, and activity has been recommended as a stimulus for development of bones in the young and protection against increased bone decomposition for the old. Evidently the surest route to avoiding inactivity is the surest route to avoiding obesity which is a nutritionally complete vegetarian diet without excesses of fat and protein.[366]

Inadequate intake of manganese may be still another factor leading to rapid loss of existing bone structure in later years. Manganese deficiency causes various animals to develop bones of low breaking strength and low density. Rabbits on a powdered milk diet, for example, had "striking" bowing of the front legs and bones were significantly reduced in weight, density, length, breaking strength and ash content. Cattle developed weak legs when deprived of manganese; pigs showed lameness and stiffness in the legs; rabbits, cattle, pigs and rats all had low density, fragile bones which could be prevented, but not cured, with manganese supplements.[367]

It is not surprising that cow's milk was employed to effect manganese deficiency. "Self-sufficiency" of foods in manganese is obtained with a manganese level of about 150 micrograms per 100 calories and cow's milk contains less than a third of that amount. Other dairy products, eggs, common meats, white bread, fats and oils and sugar are also low in manganese so the staples of the normal U.S. diet are all wanting for manganese. The deficit could be overcome with increased intake of vegetables, whole grains, legumes (especially sprouted ones) and nuts.[368]

Diets like that of the Surinam and Bantu which consist primarily of grains and lack rich sources of calcium evidently offer better defense against bone rarification than meat-based diets, but they do not seem nearly as protective as a grain-based diet containing modest amounts of low-fat dairy foods. However, dark green leafy vegetables are superior to milk as a supplement to grain-based diets. Research shows protection against osteoporosis depends on the following:

1. An akaline-ash (rather than acid-ash) diet.
2. High calcium intake.
3. A strong Ca:P ratio and a modest level of phosphorous in the diet.
4. A modest level of dietary protein.
5. Strong levels of dietary manganese.[369]

Greens provide a strongly alkaline ash whereas milk, because much of its calcium remains unabsorbed, tends to acidify the blood. Cheeses tend to be even more acidic. As a rule greens are higher in calcium than milk and many greens are lower than milk in phosphorus also. The Ca:P ratio of greens tends to be much higher than that of dairy products. The amount of protein in an ounce of greens is roughly the same as the amount in an ounce of milk, but it takes about twice as much milk as greens to obtain one's calcium needs. Higher intake means greater amounts of protein and practically speaking intake of greens is limited by their sheer bulk, whereas the amounts of milk and cheese in some diets seems to have no bounds. It has already been pointed out that milk and other dairy products are extremely poor sources of manganese. Greens are a good source.[370]

While adding greens to a whole grain-based diet is no doubt the most important step towards eliminating the threat of osteoporosis, replacing whole grains with sprouted grains and legumes promises to enhance protection even further. With sprouting the phosphorus-rich outer layer of legumes is lost and the manganese, in which grains and beans are so rich, is made readily usable.[371]

CALCULUS (STONES)

A diet designed specifically to induce calculus (kidney stones, bladder stones, etc.) in rats contains a high level of nonfat dry milk, and in a long term study of rats on a diet composed principally of dried milk, it was found that 47% of the animals developed kidney stones. Both the protein and the oil in the milk seemed to be involved, but the protein may be the main culprit for 96.7% of a group of rats given "fat-free" milk developed kidney and bladder stones. High milk intake has also been associated with stone formation in humans.[372]

Milk is very low in magnesium and lack of dietary magnesium may

be an important factor in kidney stones. Magnesium deficiency leads
to frailty, bone abnormalities and elevated serum calcium (hypercalcemia) in animals. Hypercalcemia can lead to both kidney and bladder stones, and numerous studies have shown rats developed kidney
stones when fed a low level of magnesium. The stones are often accompanied by osteoporosis. Ironically, a drug which may soon be
used to *treat* osteoporosis, acetazolamide sodium, tends to promote
kidney stones in laboratory animals.[373]

Giving humans with histories of recurring kidney stone formation
relatively small amounts of supplemental magnesium and vitamin B6
resulted in the absence of any recurrences among 30 of 36 subjects
over a period of five years. Animal studies indicate high levels of
saturated fats or high quantities of sugar sharply increase magnesium requirements, and failure to supplement high-fat or high-
sugar diets with magnesium can lead to calcium deposits in the aorta
and kidneys. Humans with calcified aortas underwent "dramatic
clinical improvement" when given a magnesium salt intrave-
nously.[374]

A review of magnesium balance done prior to 1964 led to the
conclusion magnesium intake in the U.S. was on the average less
than half of requirements and that magnesium needs are elevated by
high levels of calcium, protein, milk sugar (lactose) and vitamin
D. Most of the vitamin D in the U.S. diet is derived from vitamin
D-fortified dairy products. Most of the calcium and over a quarter of
the protein and all of the lactose in the U.S. diet is also derived from
milk and other dairy products. Unfortunately dairy products are
quite low in magnesium so that such foods, particularly fortified
milk, tend to raise calcium absorption and reduce magnesium absorption further.[375]

Nutritionists freely admit magnesium deficiency may be widespread in the U.S. but milk is only one facet of the magnesium and
stone formation problem. Meat, eggs, refined flour, sugar, fats and
oils and virtually everything else in the normal U.S. diet is painfully
low in magnesium. Whole grains, beans, peas, soybeans, dark green,
leaf vegetables and nuts are in effect the only rich sources of vitally
important magnesium. Any whole-foods vegetarian diet should offer
a plentiful supply of the mineral but vegan diets, especially those
rich in sprouts and green leaf vegetables (SGA-type diet) tend to be

the richest sources. Green vegetables also facilitate eliminating dairy products from the diet which is a key part of a sound defense against calculus.[376]

Gallstones are evidently rather widespread in the U.S. The formations are usually cholesterol-based deposits, and laboratory studies have shown that feeding animals high quantities of cholesterol leads to gallstones in a matter of days. Human gallstones are associated with excessive intake of saturated fats and cholesterol so that avoiding animal products is the obvious course for prevention.[377]

ARTHRITIS

One of the most painful conditions associated with bone degeneration and "aging" is arthritis, or inflammation of the joints. Joints are supplied with a lubricating fluid, called synovial fluid, that permits smooth joint motion, and the surfaces at which the bones meet the joints are faced with cartilage which aids the lubricating fluid by giving a degree of pliability to the contact surfaces. In arthritis the composition and characteristics of synovial fluid are altered, cartilage deteriorates and bone is deposited on contact surfaces.[378]

The most common form of arthritis is osteoarthritis, or degenerative joint disease, which afflicts well in excess of 10 million Americans. Its first signs are microscopic roughening of the cartilage which may begin in early adulthood. Symptoms usually commence after age 45 when large areas of cartilage are denuded from the bone surfaces in joints. Movement of joints tends to become painful and difficult as joints deteriorate and accumulate calcium deposits.[379]

The second most common form of arthritis is rheumatoid arthritis which affects additional millions of Americans. Rheumatoid arthritis involves chronic inflammation of joints and is often set off by some injury or damage (e.g. torn cartilage in the knee) to the affected area. Another form of arthritis is ankylosing spondylitis, which often affects the joints of the spine and pelvis. Still another form of arthritis is gout, which affects joints and leads to deposits in various internal organs.[380]

There seems to have been little attention given to the incidence of arthritis among population groups. However, gout has long been associated with the diet of the rich, and a study of jungle dwellers in India showed that they had a lesser incidence of collapse of the intervertebral discs than Europeans or North Americans. Ethnic differences appear to have no bearing on the findings since in the U.S. arthritic conditions among blacks are on a par with whites. The essentially vegetarian Abkhasians evidently avoid arthritis just as they avoid osteoporosis.[381]

Gout occurs when a sodium salt of uric acid is deposited in cartilage and bone. The deposits require an acid environment which implicates acid forming meat, poultry and fish. Flesh foods are implicated in gout in another way also. The principal constituent of gouty deposits, uric acid, is a by-product of purines in which fatty meats, poultry, organ meats, fatty fish and shellfish are high. Elevated serum uric acid is a characteristic of gout and purine-rich foods and high protein intake both tend to raise serum uric acid.[382]

Vegetables, fruits, grains, dairy products and nuts are all very low in purines and tend to keep blood levels of uric acid down. Loss of weight tends to lower serum uric acid levels also. Drugs which increase uric acid excretion are now being given to gout patients who either don't know dietary changes can lower serum uric acid or would rather become drug dependent than change. It would take a drug mentality to suggest the results of the two alternatives are the same.[383]

High levels of fat, like protein, may play a role in gout. Normally the synovial fluid which lubricates the joints contains only small amounts of fatty acids, cholesterol and phospholipids. In gout, and in other forms of arthritis, however, the fluid has enormous increases in these substances. Some physicians recommend cutting fat intake by more than half in gout, and the advice may be useful in all forms of arthritis.[384]

High intake of lard enhanced the development of osteoarthritis in mice. But a vegetable oil was found to be less injurious. The lard diet resulted in a high degree of obesity in the animals and obesity is associated with a high incidence of osteoarthritis in humans. In another study, it was found rats experienced no increase in osteoarthritis when given a lard supplement which was insufficient to produce obesity. However there seems to be a link between animal products and arthritis in humans which does not depend on obesity. Patients with pronounced arthritis exhibit elevated serum cholesterol levels, and individuals who have arthritis often have severe atherosclerosis in the aorta. It can hardly be a coincidence that cholesterol-rich nodes or knots are often seen near arthritic joints.[385]

Atherosclerosis develops rapidly in monkeys fed a diet high in cholesterol and deficient in vitamin B6, and a Texas physician found B6 to be effective in relieving the pain, stiffness and other symptoms of arthritis. Increasing intake of pantothenic acid may also aid arthritis victims for the level of pantothenic acid in the blood of arthritic patients tends to be low. Anemia is common in rheumatoid arthritis and ankylosing spondylitis, and while the anemia does not usually respond to iron it was found that folic acid did improve the anemic state of a group of rheumatoid arthritics. Riboflavin levels tend to be low in arthritis, further suggesting the B-complex plays a vital role in protection against joint degeneration.[386]

Evidently a diet which is low in lipids, especially animal fats and cholesterol and which is not heavy laden with protein but which does contain a rich supply of the B vitamins should afford strong protection against arthritis. To these ends, the SGA diet is an excellent choice. Most vegetarian diets, especially vegan ones, tend to be low in fat and cholesterol and do not carry a heavy excess of protein. Vegetarian diets also tend to be rich in folic acid and much higher in pantothenic acid than the normal U.S. diet. Normally, though, vegetarian diets are not exceptional sources of vitamin B6 or riboflavin. But the SGA diet is. And not only is it rich in B6 and riboflavin, but it contains exceptionally large amounts of folic acid and pantothenic acid. Moreover, the SGA diet contains no cholesterol, and its fat content is only a third of many vegetarian diets (and a tenth of normal U.S. diets).[387]

It is not surprising arthritis is widespread in the U.S. The U.S. diet is dominated by fat, particularly animal fat and it contains a multiple of protein needs. It also contains a heavy dose of cholesterol, and it is pathetically low in vitamin B6, pantothenic acid and folic acid.[388]

PSORIASIS

Adults with arthritis often develop a skin disease called psoriasis which involves sharply outlined, dull red patches on the skin. Psoriasis is also associated with a thickening of skin and a heavy, silvery scale. The condition is a highly chronic one which actually affects individuals of all ages as do most manifestations of aging.[389]

Exposure to sunlight tends to benefit psoriasis sufferers and (presumably) based on the widely accepted premise that any treatment should be employed that has not been proven to be harmful, physicians once used x-ray therapy to treat psoriasis. A therapy employing extensive exposure to ultra-violet rays is currently being employed. It should be interesting to hear what its proponents have to say about the relationships between exposure between ultra-violet rays and leukemia and skin cancer.[390]

The relationship between arthritis and psoriasis suggests mammalian meat, eggs and fat may be involved in the onset of psoriasis, and three physicians at Mount Sinai School of Medicine caused a stir when they replaced the usual flesh foods in the diets of 12 psoriasis patients with turkey. Ten of the twelve patients responded favorably to the switch from mammalian flesh to turkey and seven of the ten cases had "excellent response." Upon resumption of their former diet, the disease became worse, but when the turkey diet was again introduced, the disease was completely cleared.[391]

It occured to the Mount Sinai researchers that something in turkey must prevent psoriasis until they noted adding turkey to the normal diets of patients brought about no change. At this point they introduced the theory that low levels of the amino acid tryptophan cured psoriasis. Two other physicians then undermined this hypothesis when they found three psoriasis patients did not respond to low trytophan diets and pointed out that turkey is not low in tryptophan.[392]

Actually the Mount Sinai researchers were probably not far from the truth when they speculated there was something in mammalian meat that is not in turkey that causes psoriasis. It is hardly possible to interpret their clinical findings in any other way. But if this be the case, the investigators have identified mammalian meat and/or eggs as one of the, if not the only, cause of psoriasis.[393]

VISION AND HEARING

Loss of vision among aging Americans and Europeans usually results from cataracts which consist of opaque calcium-based deposits in the lens of the eye. Calcium chloride caused cataracts in cattle and low blood calcium has been implicated in human cataracts. Low serum calcium can result from kidney failure in which both excess protein and excess salt have been implicated. There is evidence that the sodium in salt may play a direct role in the development of cataracts. Injecting sodium ions into the lens of deceased humans resulted in rising opacification. The sodium invasion was accompanied by the exodus of potassium, and it was noted that the already high incidence of cataracts in the progeny of rats fed a vitamin E-deficient diet was increased when the maternal rats were given a diet high in sodium and low in potassium.[394]

From the foregoing, it is clear that vitamin E-deficient female rats tend to breed cataract-prone offspring. The embryo of hens fed a vitamin E-deficient diet tend to develop cataracts also. The question of whether the children of women taking a vitamin E-deficient diet are cataract prone has not been studied. But children can be born with cataracts and the vitamin E levels of common dietary items is exceedingly low (*see vitamin E in Appendix 4*). More to the point is the question of whether vitamin E can aid in preventing cataracts. Even if it does not, there is strong evidence that replacing dairy products, which are poor sources of vitamin E, with leaf vegetables, which are excellent sources of vitamin E, would enhance cataract defense.[395]

Dairy products are the sole dietary source of the simple sugar, galactose (milk sugar contains galactose which is freed in digestion) and high galactose diets are commonly used to produce cataracts in laboratory animals. Low-riboflavin intake speeds the development of galactose-induced cataracts but supplemental riboflavin does not prevent cataracts in galactose-fed rats and riboflavin deficiency alone evidently causes no cataracts. Galactose has also been implicated in human cataracts, and there is evidence of rising susceptibility to "galactose cataracts" with age.[396]

Galactose is not the only sugar implicated in cataracts. Cataracts have been linked to sucrose (table sugar) in animals and man, and it has been observed that placing lens in various sugars mixed with a carbohydrate known as sorbitol renders the lens opaque. The body tends to produce a large quantity of sorbitol when blood sugar is elevated and cataract formation tends to be enhanced by increased production of sorbitol. High blood sugar is, of course, a symptom of diabetes, and elderly persons with diabetes show a strong tendency to develop cataracts. Changes in the retina of the eyes and impaired vision are in fact common in diabetics of all ages.[397]

Excess food intake led to obesity, high blood sugar and cataracts in rats. Since obesity and diabetes are closely related and both conditions have been associated with a high level of fat in the diet, it is· significant that elevated serum cholesterol has been observed in senile cataract patients.[398]

Seemingly anything which pollutes the blood can adversely affect vision or initiate cataract formation. The vision of almost all of a group of patients with diseased optic nerves was improved considerably when they were given blood transfusions. The vision of alcoholics tends to be poorer than that of the overall populace, and women who take oral contraceptives are inviting vision defects. The antibiotic, streptomycin, can cause vision defects and agricultural chemicals have been linked to cataracts.[399]

The list of substances implicated in impaired hearing reads like a replay of causes of vision impairments. Sugar and fat are implicated through the tendency of diabetics to experience loss of hearing. Fat is associated with vascular disorders which apparently play a vital role in hearing defects, and it has been noted that when subjects are fed diets lower than normal in fat, especially saturated fat, over long periods, they experience improved hearing as well as a lower incidence of coronary heart disease. Antibiotics seem to affect hearing even more than vision: the use of streptomycin in 200 cases of pulmonary tuberculosis resulted in 127 cases of impaired hearing, most of them quite severe. The effects of streptomycin and other antibiotics on hearing is almost always chronic, that is permanent.[400]

Galactose (from dairy products), sodium (from salt), sugar (from a myriad of processed foods), high fat intake (especially from animal products), vitamin E deficiency, low riboflavin intake, drugs, chemicals in food and possibly excess protein have all been implicated in cataracts and impaired vision. Sugar, fat and drugs have been associated with impaired hearing. Milk and other dairy products, which provide the sole sources of galactose, are high in fat and low in vitamin E and thus should be the first items needing elimination from a diet for protection against eye and ear degeneration. Leaf vegetables, which are better calcium sources than milk, contain no galactose, little fat and high levels of vitamin E and riboflavin, afford a suitable replacement for the milk and dairy items. Meat and other animal products are high in total fats and saturated fats and thus should be cut down or excluded also. Replacing flesh products with sprouted beans and grains would add considerably to vitamin E and riboflavin intakes while lowering fat levels dramatically. Sugar clearly has no place in an anticataract diet; sugar can and should be replaced by fruits and vegetables. The advantages of a sprout-green mix are likely to be seen and heard for years to come.[401]

DIGESTION

By age 40, over a third of all Americans are believed to be afflicted with a disease known as diverticulosis, in which pressure builds up in the lower digestive tract and the walls of the large intestine thicken. The disease derives its name from the appearance of small sacs, or diverticula, along the intestine walls. Two thirds of those over 80 years of age are estimated to suffer from the disease, and some observers are beginning to regard diverticulosis as a problem common to all Westerners.[402]

Diverticulosis is associated with persistent constipation, bleeding, gastric discomfort and abdominal pain. Many sufferers experience repeated attacks during which the intestine becomes inflamed and bleeding increases. With only television commercials for a guide, the elderly often turn to the use of what therapeutic nutritionists openly call "harmful" laxatives and mineral oil to relieve constipation, and all too often victims resort to having major segments of their intestines removed by senseless surgery.[403]

Constipation is associated with failure to include adequate amounts of vitamin R, or fiber, in the diet. It has been known for many years that vitamin R stimulates peristalsis (intestinal motion) so that intestinal contents can move freely into the lower bowel. Researchers have found individuals taking the normal U.S. diet had a vitamin R intake of only a quarter that of vegetarians and low vitamin R intake may be responsible for not only recurring constipation, but diverticulosis itself.[404]

Only recently did two physicians have the foresight to prescribe a high-residue (vitamin R-rich) diet for diverticular disease, and the break from tradition proved richly rewarding. When the two doctors put 62 diverticular patients on a diet in which vitamin R was supplied in grain bran, the symptoms of 85% of the patients disappeared completely. And judging from animal studies, the treatment might have been even more effective if the whole grain had been used rather than a grain extract in the form of bran. A number of scientists now believe the lack of fiber in Western diets has changed the nature of the bacteria in the intestines to a point where a host of disorders ranging from appendicitis to bowel cancer can occur. Evidently "aging" as it pertains to the principal digestive disorder, is nothing more than too much vitamin R-deficient meat, eggs, white bread, fat, sugar and convenience items in lieu of vitamin-R rich beans, whole grains, vegetables and fruit.[405]

Hemorrhoids, or piles, is one of the most common of all "medical problems." The disease involves swellings at the lowest part of the bowel brought on by repeated dilation of the veins supplying blood to the lower bowel. The condition is believed to be caused by irregular bowel movements, constipation, continuous strenuous muscular activity and pregnancy. Thus any factor which facilitated regular bowel evacuation without strains would be expected to prevent most cases of hemorrhoids. Vitamin R, or roughage, is precisely such a factor: the vitamin as noted stimulates intestinal mobility and assures one of easy, regular evacuation.[406]

At the point where the small intestines empty into the large intestines is a pouch-like enlargement to which is attached a wormlike "cul-de-sac" two inches or more in length called the appendix.[407]

Intestinal contents may work their way into the appendix and be prevented from being expelled by inadequate peristalsis, by a blockage of the opening into the intestines, by hard fecal accumulations or by a swelling of the wall of the tract. All four of these conditions are related to intestinal stagnation which is the inevitable result of diets low in vitamin R. There is every reason to believe whole-plant food diets will facilitate the rapid expulsion of any matter entering the appendix. The inability of the appendix to empty itself leads to appendicitis which involves increased pressure and swelling in the area. As distension increases vessels may be closed off and result in gangrene. Like many victims of diverticular disease and hemorrhoids, appendicitis sufferers are forced to turn to surgery—forced by the simple lack of whole-plant foods in their diets.[408]

Peptic ulcers are a condition in which surface tissue is lost from one or more areas of the lining of the stomach or the duodenum (section of the small intestines leading from the stomach). In an advanced state additional layers of the lining of the digestive tract may be affected. Duodenal ulcers are five to ten times more common than gastric (stomach) ulcers, but gastric ulcers tend to result in more fatalities.[409]

The cells lining the stomach secrete a fluid called gastric juice which contains hydrochloric acid and an enzyme which facilitates protein digestion. Gastric juice is capable of digesting all living tissue, including the walls of the digestive tract, so that the body must provide protection for the walls of the stomach and duodenum. Protection depends on the secretion of mucus by the stomach, on dilution and neutralization of the gastric juice by injested food and on saliva from the mouth. Western diets tend to promote ulcers by promoting excess secretion of gastric juice and causing a high concentration of hydrochloric acid in the gastric juice. Normal Western diets also tend to reduce protection against gastric acidity.[410]

Gastric juice secretion is stimulated by a hormone known as gastrin and an inordinate rise in the level of calcium in the blood tends to affect a rise in serum gastrin, hence production of an excess of gastric juice. Elevated serum calcium usually results from decalcification of the bones though it can be brought on by an excess of dietary calcium.[411]

Since bone decalcification is likely to be the result of excessive intake of acid ash forming "protein" in foods, especially meat and eggs, animal products become a prime suspect in the overproduction of gastric juice. There is a strong possibility of an even more direct tie between high serum gastrin and meat. Meats, especially blood-rich meats, are exceptionally high in the amino acid histidine. In the body much of the histidine is converted into a related substance known as histamine which may be identical to gastric juice production stimulating gastrin.[412]

When high serum gastrin is brought on by an excess of dietary calcium, it is almost certain to be the result of high milk intake or calcium supplements. Ulcer patients are frequently advised to take large quantities of milk, and they are often given supplementary calcium. The purpose of these recommendations is to neutralize the gastric juice, but any true gain may be offset by the tendency of rising serum calcium to elevate gastric acid excretion.[413]

Fortunately there are foods which tend to neutralize gastric juice acidity without increasing gastric juice output. Particularly effective are members of the cabbage family which include green, leafy vegetables like turnip greens and mustard greens. So effective in reducing gastric acidity of ulcer patients is a sulfur-containing substance found in members of the cabbage family that the substance has been designated as "vitamin U." Ulcer patients and those wishing to avoid ulcers can not rely on intermittent intake of leafy vegetables for vitamin U, however. Studies with laboratory animals indicate there is almost no vitamin U stored by the body and therefore it is necessary to make these leafy vegetables a regular item in the diet if constant protection is desired.[414]

Western physicians recognize the value of vegetables and other plant foods in treating ulcers. They even recognize the dangers of meat, eggs, salt, fats, alcohol, coffee and smoking in ulcers. It is unfortunate they only recommend abstention from these killers *after* the walls of the digestive tract are damaged.[415]

Caffeine and aspirin both tend to produce ulcers in animals and man. Smoking threatens the integrity of the walls of the gastrointestinal tract and like meat, stimulates the overproduction of gastric juice. Western diets as a whole tend to raise the acidity of saliva so that one of the vital mechanisms by which the body protects the stomach and duodenum from gastric acidity is impaired. Highly seasoned foods of any kind tend to aggravate ulcers.[416]

The SGA diet contains none of the specific foods implicated in causing peptic ulcers, and the large quantity of greens in the SGA diet provide an abundant supply of protective vitamin U. The complete spectrum of vitamins, minerals and other necessary nutrients contained in the SGA mix offers the strongest possible assurance of a sound, efficient digestive system. The SGA diet also provides a strong buffering capacity to protect against the acidity of gastric juice and to prevent overproduction of the juice. And since the SGA diet is also very rich in vitamin R, it promises the strongest possible defenses against digestive disorders in general.[417]

SUMMARY AND CONCLUSIONS

Animal foods have been implicated in every aspect of "aging." Animal products in general, and meat in particular, stimulate rapid growth and large body size, characteristics which are direct paths to reduced life span and high incidence of degenerative disease in animals. The world's longest-living and most disease-free inhabitants take almost no meat or other flesh foods and the magnificent Hunzas are in essence, total vegetarians.[418]

Animal products tend to produce a high degree of acidity in the blood which promotes osteoporosis by forcing the bones to give up calcium as a buffering media. All animal foods are high in phosphorus and protein both of which have been implicated directly in bone decalcification. Flesh foods themselves cause rapid bone loss and poor bone development in animals and deteriorating bones in humans. Humans tend to experience rapid bone losses when they are inactive over an extended period, and animal products promote poor endurance in athletes and seem to have left inhabitants of North America and Europe in a state of enjoying nothing more than doing nothing.[419]

All animal products are very poor sources of manganese and magnesium. Manganese deficiency causes severe underdevelopment of bone structure in various animals and low intake of magnesium results in poor bone development, calcium-based kidney stones and atherosclerotic deposits in animals. So poor is cow's milk in manganese that animals are given diets rich in cow's milk to study the effects of manganese deficiency (and poor bone development). Cow's milk has also been implicated in kidney stones and humans with recurrent kidney stones have benefited from increased magnesium intake. Dietary cholesterol induces gall bladder stones in animals and animal products have been implicated in the condition in humans.[420]

Arthritis has been closely linked to atherosclerosis and obesity. Atherosclerosis is, of course, related to excesses of animal fats and (animal derived) cholesterol while obesity has been linked to animal fats and protein. Osteoarthritis has been induced in laboratory animals with animal fat and high protein levels; fat and cholesterol are involved in gout, which is a form of arthritis. Milk and common meats are poor sources of folacin and vitamin B6 which may aid arthritic patients. Psoriasis, which often occurs with arthritis, has been linked to intake of certain animal products also. [421]

High intake of milk sugar leads to rapid development of cataracts in animals and high fat levels have been implicated in impairment of both sight and hearing in humans. Vitamin E deficiency may be involved in cataract formation and animal products are invariably low in vitamin E. [422]

Animal products contain virtually no roughage, or vitamin R, which is the key to a sound digestive tract. Constipation and hemorrhoids are taken as normal in the U.S., and most Americans who reach retirement age have developed an advanced state of diverticular disease. The latter has been cured in many cases by simply giving patients the vitamin R of whole grains. Hemorrhoids and appendicitis are also linked to the lack of vitamin R and excesses of animal products and lack of green vegetables. Acid-forming flesh foods set the stage for ulcers while green vegetables protect against the symptoms and causes of ulcers. [423]

Thus animal products have been implicated in reduced life spans, poor bone development and skeletal degeneration, osteoporosis, stone formation, arthritis, psoriasis, impaired vision and hearing, digestive disorders and of course, atherosclerosis. Not to mention cancer, obesity, diabetes, multiple sclerosis, kidney failure, liver disorders and emotional distresses which are not in the definitional sense aspects of "aging." For those who choose to live full, long, outgoing lives, the message should be clear: stop eating meat, eggs and dairy products. [424]

Giving up animal products is not the whole answer of course. Refined carbohydrates, especially sugar, have been implicated in reduced life spans, osteoporosis and stones (through manganese and magnesium deficiencies), arthritis, diverticular disease, cataracts and atherosclerosis. Salt, medicines and stimulants have also been implicated in "aging." What normal diets need is a complete rejection. [425]

A suitable beginning for a new diet is raw sprouts of soybeans and legumes serving as acid-free sources of protein, magnesium, manganese, folic acid, vitamin B6, vitamin R, vitamin E and a host of other nutrients. But a sound diet needs a strong calcium source and the best sources are the dark green, leaf vegetables like raw collard greens, rutabaga greens and parsley. Greens add rich amounts of a broad range of nutrients including all of those associated with preventing some facet of aging. A mix of sprouts and greens offers a good supply of all the necessary vitamins and minerals with the possible exceptions of iodine and vitamin B_{12}, but a little algae, as seaweed or in some other form, can fill in with iodine and B_{12}. The resulting SGA mix is a vital alternative to aging.[426]

5 / protein

PART 1: PROTEIN FOR BODY MAINTENANCE NEEDS

Next to water, protein composes the greatest proportion of the body tissues, and tissue proteins are in a continuous state of change. Tissue is constantly casting off protein which, upon being discarded, is disassembled into its component amino acids (the nitrogen-containing building blocks of protein). Dietary protein is also broken down into its component amino acids before being absorbed. Upon entering the bloodstream the newly absorbed amino acids become mixed with the amino acids from dismantled tissue proteins to form a pool of amino acids available for (1) reassembly as body proteins, (2) for use as an energy source and (3) for breakdown into products of excretion.[427]

It is estimated that half the body's tissue protein is cast off in only three months. So dynamic is protein turnover that the body's pool of amino acids normally affords less than two weeks' requirements for synthesis of new protein alone. However, the rate of turnover is not independent of protein intake. On a protein-free diet, the rate of breakdown of tissue protein and synthesis of new protein may slip to a third of normal. When, on the other hand, protein intake is raised to three times needs as it is in typical Western diets, the breakdown of tissue protein may be doubled. A sense of well-being accompanies the metabolic bonfire set off by the ingestion of a large quantity of protein, and the "rush" has led many individuals to believe high protein intake brings surging health: it is best that they remember that sugar, coffee, cigarettes, alcohol and hard drugs also give rushes and that runaway protein synthesis is the essence of cancer.[428]

What the average person "knows" about protein is worse than nothing because for the most part it is false and it can lead to harmful practices. Popular misconceptions about protein include the following:[429]

1. *The more protein you eat the better.* Nothing could be further from the truth. There is nothing to be gained by an excess of protein. High protein intake has been implicated in such diverse disorders as kidney failure, gout, osteoporosis, breast cancer, bowel cancer, cancer of the pancreas, liver cirrhosis, obesity, reduced life expectancy, atherosclerosis and lack of endurance.[430]

2. *Meat, eggs and cheese are "protein foods."* It is more accurate to classify these items as "fat foods" for they derive an average of about 70% of their calories from fats. Fat and fat-related components of meat, eggs and cheese have tied them in the strongest possible way to all of the major degenerative diseases including cardiovascular disease, cancer, diabetes, arthritis, obesity and multiple sclerosis. Almost all of the nonfat calories of meat, eggs and many cheeses are indeed derived from protein but this only strengthens the tendency for these foods to reduce life expectancy, promote obesity, cancer, gout, atherosclerosis and various other disorders.[431]

3. *You need more protein when you do hard physical work.* This is utterly false. Over 50 years of research with humans has repeatedly demonstrated the most strenuous types of activity cause no increase in need for protein.[432]

4. *Protein builds endurance.* Again the public has been misled. High carbohydrate diets are the key to increased physical endurance and high-fat, high-protein animal products tend to reduce endurance.[433]

5. *High-protein diets are the best way to lose weight.* The only way to lose weight and keep weight down is to choose a diet which achieves lower weight and to stick with that diet. While lean-meat diets have effected weight losses for some, they have devastating side effects that can only lead to early degeneration. Strict vegetarian diets have resulted in more consistent and more rapid weight losses, and people who stay on vegetarian diets remain slim while lean-meat dieters almost always regain lost weight as soon as they return to their normal ways of eating.[434]

6. *Wounds heal faster with high protein intake.* Again, research refutes the popular belief. Elevated protein intake does nothing to speed wound healing or protein losses associated with injury or surgery.[435]

7. *Protein deficiency is widespread*. At best this statement is grossly misleading. A major segment of the world's population is indeed underfed, but if the underfed were provided with enough grains, beans and vegetables to supply their nonprotein needs, few, if any, would require more protein. It is possible to get enough calories without getting enough protein but one needs help from the food processors to achieve that unhappy state: sugar, alcoholic beverages, fats and oils and other refined foods are just about the only clearly protein-deficient foods.[436]

8. *Babies certainly need a high level of protein*. Most untrue. For infants, there is a perfect food: human milk. And human milk derives only about 7% of calories from protein. That's about a third as much as cow's milk and puts human milk behind all grains, beans and vegetables in protein content.[437]

9. *Vegetarian diets may lead to protein deficiency*. This is one of the most misleading statements one could possibly make about protein. Vegetarian diets based on grains, beans, soybeans and vegetables are second to none in providing strong amounts of good quality protein. A diet loaded with sugar, oil, alcohol and fruit would, of course, be deficient in just about everything, including protein. It is indeed sound advice to warn all people to avoid sugar, oil and alcohol; it's unfortunate defenders of the normal diet do not offer such advice.[438]

Several of these disclaimers were substantiated in previous chapters, but for clarity they will be given at least cursory attention again in this chapter. The present chapter will also offer substantiation of the foregoing disclaimers that have not been discussed previously and deal with other aspects of dietary protein.[439]

PROTEIN REQUIREMENTS

Studies with young adults indicate that theoretical needs for protein total about 25 grams of protein per day for men weighing under 175 pounds and less than 20 grams of protein per day for normal women. However, such protein levels would not be adequate unless the protein were very efficient in the sense it caused no increase in excretory losses of nitrogen. This would rarely, if ever, be the case since no protein is likely to be 100% absorbed and unabsorbed protein increases fecal nitrogen. Moreover, the protein absorbed may alter the body's pool of amino acids so as to cause at least some increase in urinary nitrogen.[440]

It was long believed egg protein was the most efficient protein in the sense that the amount of egg protein required for "maintenance," that is, to compensate for excretory losses of nitrogen, was less than the amount for any other protein. However, recent studies in Germany have shown the protein of potatoes is as efficient as egg protein and suggest that common food mixes may result in proteins that are even more efficient than the protein of egg or potatoes. A mix of corn and beans was at least as efficient as potatoes or egg alone, and a mix of corn, beans and potatoes might have improved protein efficiency still further.[441]

Numerous studies have shown protein needs with single grains as the sole source of protein are less than .70 grams of protein per kilogram body weight per day. This suggests normal adults would need 30 to 55 grams of protein per day from a single grain source. It would require well over 700 grams of grain per day to match normal caloric intakes and 700 grams of millet, wheat, triticale, oats or corn would provide 66 to 100 grams of protein which means diets consisting wholly of one of these grains should provide more than adequate amounts of protein. Rice is lower in protein than other grains yet it has been shown rice alone is a totally adequate source of protein for young men. These are very important observations because the protein of single grains alone is among the most inefficient proteins known. The addition of beans and/or vegetables (especially leaf vegetables) or other plant foods to grains tends both to increase protein efficiency and boost total protein levels. A mix of grain and beans lowers protein requirements to about 0.55 grams per kilogram of body weight per day which is about 30 grams per day for a small woman and 39 grams per day for a 160-pound man. Studies with young adults accustomed to normal American-type diets have shown they adapt well to lacto-vegetarian diets and their maintenance needs (which constitute the total protein requirements of adults) are satisfied with 40 grams of protein per day. Rarely do even strict vegetarian diets provide less than 60 grams of protein per day. Studies involving young adults on strict vegetarian diets show intakes of only 45 grams of protein per day are above maintenance requirements.[442]

The foregoing makes it clear that protein needs, regardless of the nature of the protein, are much lower than most people realize. However, these findings should be taken in context since studies on protein requirements are almost always conducted in the presence of normal caloric intakes. A survey of maintenance requirement studies done prior to 1954 suggested no amount of protein was likely to be adequate for adults taking fewer than 1500 calories per day. Subsequently, though, two British scientists discovered that the protein needs of obese young adults on diets providing only 1000 calories per day could be satisfied by doubling their protein intake. The British researchers also found that the protein requirements of rats restricted to 40% of their customary calorie intake could be met when protein constituted a very high 40% of the animal's diet.[443]

Even modest reductions in calorie intake tend to elevate protein needs. Investigators found the protein needs of young men rose substantially when their caloric intake was lowered by only 20%. As might be expected an excess of calories tends to reduce protein requirements. In a study involving 28 male students over a two-year period, it was found a 25% excess of calories lowers the requirements for egg protein by 30% and the (higher) need for rice protein by 50%. Thus the requirements for what are usually regarded as poor quality proteins may actually be less than the requirements for the most heralded proteins when the former are accompanied by higher caloric intakes. The crown once worn by egg protein has been twice tarnished.[444]

Exhibit P1 is an effort to graph the relationship between caloric intake and protein requirements for adults. The unbroken curve is an estimate of protein needs versus calories when the protein is a fairly efficient one. It is based on five separate studies. The broken line is based on two studies and is an estimate of protein needs at various caloric levels when the protein is derived from a single grain alone.[445]

A survey of U.S. households in 1957 indicated the average American was taking over 60 calories per kilogram of body weight. From Exhibit P1 it appears such an intake would bring down protein needs to less than 3% of calories, but the 1957 survey showed individuals were actually deriving 13% of their calories from protein which evidently amounts to more than four times their actual needs.[446]

Strict vegetarian diets which are free of processed foods almost always provide more than 10% of calories as protein. Some provide over 20% of calories as protein. From Exhibit P1 it can be seen that diets

Protein Requirements for Maintenance as Function of Calories

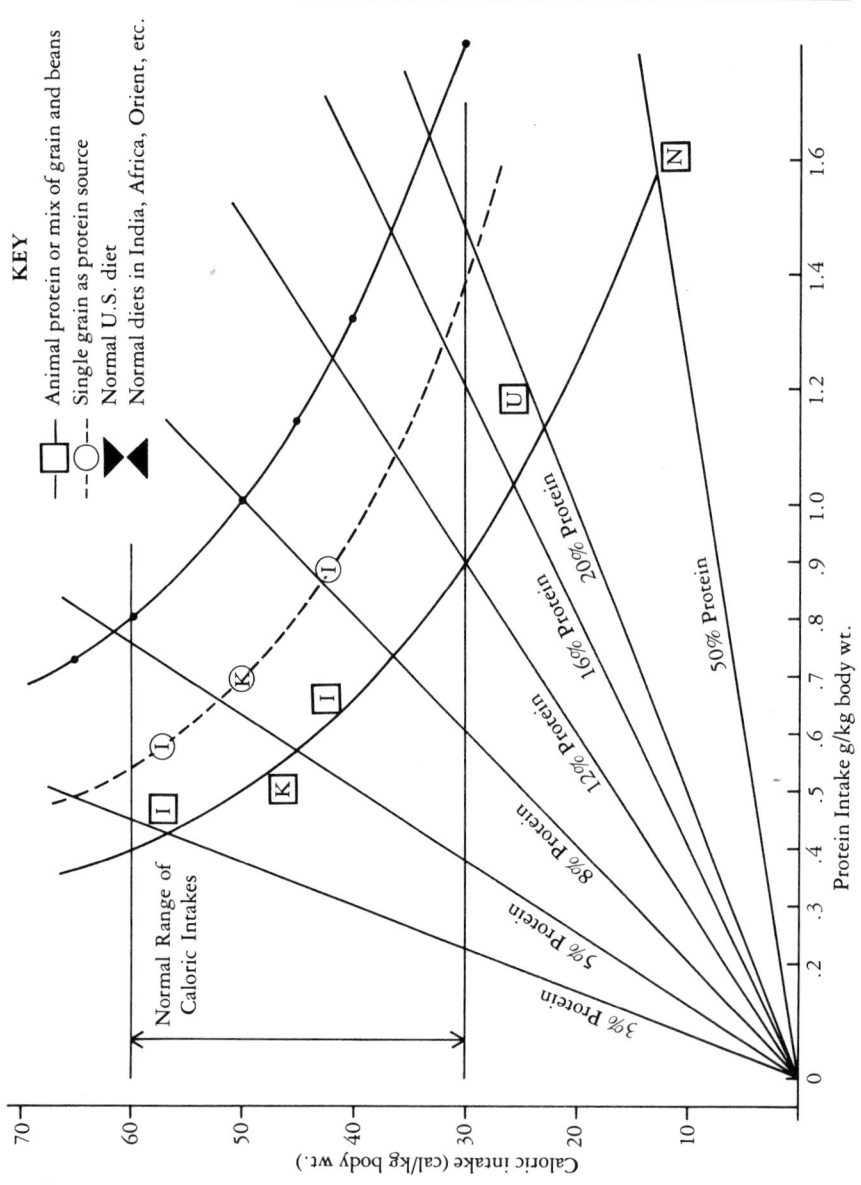

Sources   I = Inoue, G. et al. J.Nutr., 103(12):1673, 1973.
           K = Kofranye, E., et al. Hoppe-Sylers Z. Physol Chem., 351(12): 1485,
               1970.
           N = Naismeth, D.J. and Holdsworth, M.D. Proc. Nutr. Soc., 29(2):
               55A, 1970.
           U = USAF Air Mtl. Command Reports No. 5740 and MCREXD–691–
               3H, 1948.

containing 10% protein require energy intakes of 30 to 40 calories per kilogram for positive nitrogen balance. This amounts to less than 2300 calories per day for an average sized woman and under 3000 calories per day for most men. Thus there seems to be no danger of protein deficiency for adults who avoid processed foods.[447]

Hard work and exercise cause no increase in protein needs. It has been shown repeatedly that protein combustion is no higher during heavy exercise than under resting conditions. Exercising muscles normally exhaust available carbohydrate stores before turning to other energy sources, and it has been found that even after exhaustion of the carbohydrate deposits, continued exercise does not boost protein requirements significantly. When rats are induced to increase their activity levels by feeding them a calorically restricted diet they lose body fat but they retain almost all of their body protein. This reflects an actual decrease in protein needs during exercise for when caloric intake is restricted and the animals are forced to remain idle, they use up sizeable amounts of protein. Athletes performing endurance tasks and burning up to 9000 calories per day show no noticeable increase in protein needs.[448]

When it became clear that heavy work per se does not increase protein needs some observers warned sweat losses of nitrogen might still result in higher protein needs during heavy work in hot environments. But when researchers put six young Jamaicans on heavy exercise routines during successive five-day periods, they found total protein needs did not increase at all. The subjects spent seven hours per day in the tropical sun clearing brush, playing football, cycling, etc., during which time they lost over six pints of sweat per day. But their sweat was relatively low in nitrogen and their urinary excretion of nitrogen fell to compensate for sweat losses. The subjects were in positive nitrogen balance with protein intakes of less than 50 grams per day.[449]

Endurance tends to decrease as protein intake is elevated. It was found a high-protein diet led to reduced build-ups in muscle carbohydrate and lower endurance times on a bicycle ergmeter than did high-carbohydrate diets. Distance runners took 143 minutes to traverse a 19-mile course on the standard "mixed" (meat-rich) diet. With a high-carbohydrate diet their muscle carbohydrate increased and they cut their running time to 135 minutes. A pair of Russian researchers advocated high-carbohydrate diets for athletes in training, suggesting high protein intake only during periods of inactivity. It is interesting that rats on a "protein deficient" diet were smaller than controls, but when forced to run to exhaustion they ran an average of over seven hours while controls lasted just over four hours. As indicated above rats tend to increase activity levels when deprived of protein or calories though high-fat intake sharply reduces the increased activity resulting from a protein-free diet.[450]

There is typically an increase in urinary nitrogen excretion following injury, and it was once thought that protein intake should be elevated during recovery from injury. However, it was subsequently found that even extremely high protein intakes did not prevent the transient rise in nitrogen losses following injury. A team of researchers headed by the eminent nutritionist, Dr. Doris Callaway lent support to the belief that neither injury nor surgery boost protein needs when they found animals fed three times as much protein as normal recovered no better from wounds than those fed only normal amounts of protein.[451]

Living at high altitudes causes no increase in protein needs. Indeed cutting protein intake may enhance cell respiration at high altitudes for it was found arterial oxygen was increased by raising carbohydrate intake at 11,000 feet and that high-protein diets depressed the growth of rats at high altitudes. High fat also depressed growth, though not as severely as high protein.[452]

By now it should be clear that adults do not need high levels of protein. Any calorically adequate whole-foods diet that is not dominated by fruit offers an abundant amount of protein and neither hard work, hot climates, injury nor high altitudes boost protein needs. Normal Western diets provide a multiple of maintenance needs so it is important to consider the implications of excess protein.[453]

THE EFFECTS OF HIGH PROTEIN INTAKE

As noted above endurance tends to decline as protein intake is elevated. Overweight individuals are characteristically inactive, and a sizable segment of the world's total supply of natural resources is being rushed into making it possible for the heavy-protein eaters of the world to avoid any semblance of physical activity. In a very real sense virtually everyone in the protein-rich nations is obese for individuals in those areas who weigh 20% to 30% less than the average enjoy longer life expectancies and lower incidences of cardiovascular disease, cancer, diabetes, hypertension and numerous other degenerative disorders.[454]

There is growing evidence high protein intake plays a major role in obesity. For many years nutritionists sought to assure the public that high fat intake had little or nothing to do with obesity. They based this incredible claim on research with laboratory animals who showed little tendency to become obese on relatively high-fat, low-protein diets. It is only when animals were put on high-fat diets which also contained fairly high amounts of protein that animals began to develop such marked obesity that they looked as wide as they did long. The amounts of fat and protein necessary to double the amount of fat in rats and mice were no more than one gets in a T-bone steak.[455]

Examination of the excess body tissue of obese mice showed the tissue contained significantly more protein than the tissues of non-obese mice, and one group of researchers found the food intake of rats on high-protein diets had to be restricted in order to prevent them from gaining more weight than rats taking normal diets. Two British scientists reported high protein alone led to obesity in rats. The addition of a high level of fat to the high-protein diet led to more pronounced obesity, and that is just how Westerners get most of their protein—with lots of fat. The clear message from studies of obesity in animals is that high-carbohydrate diets are the key to avoiding obesity.[456]

It is ludicrous to label "starchy" foods as fattening. The Kempner rice diet has been used for decades, and even when eaten in unrestricted quantity, it usually results in substantial weight losses. Under controlled conditions it was found a low-protein, low-calorie diet gave excellent results in treating obesity, and a calorically unrestricted high-carbohydrate, low-protein diet was highly effective in treating obese patients. Weight losses averaged about two pounds per week on the high-carbohydrate diet. The SGA diet which puts no restriction on the amount of potatoes, has been 100% effective in achieving rapid weight losses among obese individuals.[457]

The effectiveness of low-protein, high-carbohydrate diets in treating obesity should not be surprising. Anyone who has visited the Orient, Africa, Latin America, India or the Middle East has been exposed to the fact that high-carbohydrate diets result in slim body frames. The obesity one encounters in those regions occurs among businessmen, politicians and others who have joined the animal fat and protein feast. The slimness resulting from low-fat, low-protein diets can also be seen in vegetarians in the meat-eating regions. Studies show that as the degree of vegetarianism increases, average body weight decreases. Perhaps there is an obese strict vegetarian somewhere on earth, but the author has yet to meet one.[458]

In the preceding chapter it was noted that high-protein diets in general and high-meat diets in particular result in rapid losses in bone calcium. Vast numbers of Americans and Europeans taking conventional diets are plagued with debilitating losses in bone structure in the form of osteoporosis. There is no evidence of osteoporosis among the essentially lacto-vegetarian Abkhasians or the almost totally vegetarian Hunzas.[459]

Protein tends to acidify the blood thereby forcing bones to give up calcium to buffer the acidity. A series of studies with groups of young men at the University of Wisconsin have shown high protein intake causes rapid loss of bone calcium whereas low protein intake prevents bone deterioration. The same association between high protein intake and bone degeneration has been demonstrated in animals, and years of work with human subjects at the University of California make it clear that high protein intake increases the amount of calcium excreted. It is all too clear that high protein intake tends to cause deterioration of the body frame.[460]

High-protein, high-fat diets have been advocated for rapid growth, which indeed they foster. The height of two-year-olds today is three to four inches above that of two-year-olds 70 years ago, and weights are proportionally greater. It is reported that high-fat and high-protein diets are 20% more effective than high-carbohydrate diets in promoting growth and accelerating physical development. That high-fat and high-protein diets may reduce activity levels seems to have been dismissed by observers who regard exercise as a "stress factor" that may "hinder physical development." Perhaps exercise does place a stress on persons taking excessive amounts of protein and fat, but this hardly alters the fact that individuals taking milder diets give every sign of enjoying and benefiting from physical activity.[461]

The objectives of rapid growth and accelerated development are incompatible to long life and resistance to degenerative disease. Cancer researchers report dietary regimes leading to rapid structural and biochemical growth rates are detrimental to health and lead to marked reductions in life expectancy.[462]

In a series of experiments begun a half century ago at Cornell University, Dr. Clive McCoy evaluated the effects of dietary excesses on the life span of animals. He found that white rats deprived of dietary calories and protein grew slowly, but after 1000 days, when virtually all "normal" rats were dead, the sparsely fed rats were active, alert, had glossy coats and low pulse rates and were strongly resistant to disease. The few remaining "well-nourished" rats were deformed, crooked and "ill-faced, worse bodied." The slow-growing rats lived to an average age of 1400 days or double the life span of controls. The experiments were eventually extended to other animals ranging from cockroaches to brook trout and the results were always the same, rapid growth led to disease, degeneration and much shorter lifespans. Recently it was found that cutting back on dietary intake of calories, protein and fat, even at advanced age, increases the life spans of rats markedly. One-year-old rats for example have a life expectancy of less than 9 months on their normal laboratory regime but cutting their protein, fat and caloric intakes by about 40% raises their life expectancy to 14 months. Some years ago it was found feeding rats about .8 grams of protein per day, which is about a fifth of the amount that is required for maximal growth, slowed degeneration and substantially increased life span.[463]

The conclusions of a group of scientists that "Overnutrition has a bad influence on life span" and that "it is especially true with growth-promoting animal origin calories . . ." is hardly debatable. There are countries in Eastern Europe, Western Europe, North America, South America, Central America, East Asia and Oceania with lower mortality rates than those in the U.S. and Britain. So-called "undernourished" animals and men have been found more resistant to viruses, and the incidence of various cancers in animals is cut drastically by restricting food intake. The incidence, growth and spread of breast cancer, liver tumors, lymphatic malignancies and other cancers accompanies reduction in protein intake. The cancer-free, long-living Abkhasians and Hunzas have protein intakes 30% to 50% below those of Americans and Western Europeans. The Abkhasians and Hunzas seldom eat flesh foods, they grow slower and they are smaller than Americans, but they remain astoundingly active at advanced ages, avoiding not only cancer, but diabetes, hypertension, intestinal disorders and other degenerative diseases. Their aged reportedly maintain excellent eyesight, teeth and hearing.[464]

Presumably the idea that rapid growth and large size are desirable stems from work with animals when the objective was raising the profits of animal breeders. No doubt livestock breeders benefit financially from high-fat, high-protein diets by people, as well as their animals, but it is sobering to note that in a long term study, beef cattle fed the normal growth promoters developed a very high incidence of eye cancer. To be sure they were larger, heavier and grew fatter than cattle left to their own in pastures, but the slower growers were much healthier and rarely developed eye cancer.[465]

The role of protein in atherosclerosis is not clear, but the serum cholesterol levels of laboratory animals are said to correlate closely with the level of protein in their diets. Humans put on a diet containing only 25 grams of protein per day had a remarkable drop in serum cholesterol, and children given a supplement of animal or vegetable protein experienced a rise in serum cholesterol. Strict vegetarians have much lower serum cholesterol levels than meat-eaters, but it is not clear that lower protein intake is involved. The Kempner (rice) diet which provides only 15 to 30 grams of protein per day has been shown to lower serum cholesterol, but the reasons for the effect are obscured by the low fat content of the regime. In any event, antiatherosclerotic diets tend to be low in animal products. The adoption of high-protein, Western diets by immigrants from low mortality countries leads to increased mortality from coronary heart disease and intake of protein, meat and eggs parallels the incidence of atherosclerosis and degenerative heart disease.[466]

High protein intake has been implicated in uremia, a disease in which the kidneys are unable to eliminate protein wastes, particularly urea. When protein intake is high, urea production increases but when protein intake is cut or vegetable protein is substituted for animal protein, serum urea tends to fall markedly.[467]

Unless treated, uremia can be fatal and low-protein diets have been used in Italy to treat both reversible and chronic uremia. Chronic uremia can evidently be rendered symptom-free for years with diets containing only 20 grams of protein per day. The low-protein (Italian) diet brought about rapid improvement of clinical symptoms of uremia for almost all of 23 Canadian patients. The Canadian physicians who administered the diet noted it was also effective in treating other kidney disorders, even comas.[468]

The Russians have been treating chronic renal (kidney) insufficiency with a potato diet and other low-protein diets for years, and a Hungarian group reports uremic symptoms subside or disappear with diets containing 18 to 24 grams of protein. Extremely low-protein diets are, for most people, not the most palatable, and they seemingly could be avoided by abstaining from extremely high protein intakes before pathological states develop.[469]

The acid ash of protein has been implicated in kidney stones and the waste products of protein metabolism may cause precipitation of calcium phosphate to form urinary stones. High protein levels in the presence of modest amounts of fat from various oils led to gallstones in rabbits in only 12 weeks. On a lower protein intake rabbits exhibited a "marked degree of protection" from gallstones even when fat intake was increased as long as the carbohydrate in their diet consisted of rice starch rather than sugar. Cholesterol and cholic acid, in which eggs and flesh products are high, led to gallstones in mice.[470]

Foods that are high in protein are usually high in purine as well. The richest sources of purine are liver and other organ meats, fatty flesh and meat extracts. A by-product of purine metabolism is uric acid, and when blood levels of uric acid rise, deposits form in soft tissues and joints to produce gout, a form of arthritis. Uric acid is also associated with one form of kidney stones.[471]

Removing red meat and eggs from the diets of patients suffering from psoriasis, a chronic skin disease, resulted in excellent response from seven of 12 patients and only two failed to respond to the change. High levels of protein, especially milk protein, resulted in amyloidosis, a disorder affecting the spleen, liver, kidneys and other organs, in mice. An excess of the amino acid tyrosine, in which eggs and milk protein are high, resulted in corneal lesions in rats and cataracts may be related to amino acid excesses also.[472]

Studies of the relationship between calcium retention and protein intake indicate that when caloric intake is high (say 3000 calories per day for a 154 pound individual) a protein intake of 2 grams per kilogram bodyweight (140 grams per day for a 154 pounder) leads to rapid bone attrition. Bone losses apparently begin at protein levels of 1.4 to 1.9 grams per kilogram, which, from Exhibit P1, is two to three times the requirements for protein from single grains alone and three to four times the requirements on a mixed diet. While estimates of average protein intake vary, a U.S. Department of Agriculture survey put average protein levels at about 2 grams per kilogram with an average energy intake of 70 calories per kilogram, which is enough to cause bone losses in any normal adult. Whatever the actual average intake is, North Americans are taking far more protein than their bodies need; and judging by the prevalence of disorders related to protein excesses most are taking harmful excesses.[473]

There is no danger of receiving an excess of protein on the SGA diet. Protein levels would be adequate with energy intakes of 1000 to 1500 calories per day, and it is inconceivable persons would take larger amounts of the basics, that is sprouts and greens. Most persons taking the SGA diet derive fewer than 800 calories per day from sprouts and greens and obtain the remainder of their calories from comparatively low protein foods like potatoes, sweet potatoes, fruit, etc., so that protein, as a percentage of calories declines as caloric intake is increased.[474]

"PROTEIN FOODS"

Animal products, especially meat, are affectionately labeled "protein foods." It should be clear by now that if the "protein" label were justified it would hardly justify affection, and the real essence of most animal products is not protein but fat.[475]

Any item which derives more than 25% of calories from fat tends to load the diet with fat. Certainly any item deriving more than 40% of its calories from fat should be classified as "fatty." Beef derives about 75% of its calories from fat and 25% from protein; eggs get about 70% of their calories from fat and 30% from protein and milk obtains over 50% of its calories from fat with just over 20% coming from protein. Popular cheeses are roughly 70% fat and even so-called "lean meat" derives about 50% of its calories from fat. Fish and fowl tend to be considerably lower in fat than mammalian flesh, but fish, chicken, etc. are usually fried in oil, broiled with butter, or canned in oil, hence end up as fatty products also.[476]

The adverse effects of high fat when backed by high protein levels are vast, and the extremely high level of fat in so-called "protein foods" makes it appropriate to recall some of the adverse effects of high fat alone. High-fat diets shorten the life span of laboratory animals. High fat intake induces various cancers in laboratory animals and a constituent of heated animal fats produces cancer in animals. Beef and high fat have been implicated in "the most common major form of cancer in the U.S. (100,000 new cases this year)—cancer of the bowel." Dietary fat has been linked to breast cancer, which is the most prevalent cancer among women and rapidly growing pancreatic cancer. Fat has also been implicated in kidney cancer. The first American study directed at relating cancer incidence to degree of vegetarianism is now underway, and preliminary results indicate even modest reductions in dietary fat and flesh may reduce cancer mortality by 40% or more. High fat intake has been implicated in diabetes, gallstones, arthritis, multiple sclerosis and a host of other disorders. There is a vast body of data implicating high intake of total fat, animal fats and fat-related cholesterol, which occurs only in animal products, in coronary heart disease and other diseases related to atherosclerosis. Even the most conservative researchers are now calling for sharp cuts in total fat intake and drastic reductions in animal fats; some researchers go so far as recommending total elimination of "saturated fats and cholesterol-containing foods."[477]

Provided the protein level is adequate, high-fat diets produce gross obesity in animals. It has been found that the more fat that is included in diets of mice, the higher is their body fat content. Proclivity to obesity from high fat is evidently independent of strain or sex. Rats also respond to high-fat, high-protein diets with gross obesity though there seems to be the same advantage to taking vegetable oils vis-a-vis butter or lard. Obesity is not seen where individuals take little fat. Hunza males reportedly take 36 grams of fat a day compared to a 157 gram average for Americans as a whole. The perpetually slim Abkhasians take low levels of fat also.[478]

If there is one clear fact creditable to modern nutrition it is that high-fat diets, particularly when the fat is derived from animal sources, are detrimental to health. Calling meat, eggs, milk, cheese and fried chicken "protein foods" does not alter their status. They are loaded with fat of a saturated nature. People like them, it is argued. Their bodies don't, the research answers.[479]

THE POOR NATIONS

Individuals in underfed countries are receiving on the average about 35 calories per kilogram which puts their protein requirement at about .76 grams per kilogram if the protein efficiency were high and about 1.13 grams per kilogram if the protein were derived from a single grain.[480]

Unfortunately large segments of the underfed do rely on a single grain for a large proportion of their calories and protein. The average protein intake of such people is probably about .8 to .9 grams per kilogram, which is below apparent needs. *Increasing food intake would have a double-barreled tendency to wipe out any protein deficit, for it would decrease the need for protein while raising intake.* A representative of the World Health Organization of the United Nations reported that "In only one out of ten cases does protein deficiency occur as a direct result of inadequate protein intake. In the vast majority of cases protein deficiency is the result of inadequate intake of total energy." This acknowledgement may be somewhat of an understatement since it is not generally recognized that increasing caloric intake actually reduces protein needs.[481]

Recommendations to simply increase the amount of grain in grain-based diets may be impossible for many. An alternative might be increased cultivation and increased intake of soybeans or legumes and leaf vegetables at the expense of lowering grain intake. Mixing grains with beans, peas or soybeans markedly increases protein efficiency, and the addition of leaf vegetables should improve the efficiency of a grain and bean mix still further. An SGA-type mix of red spring wheat as 70% of calories, mung beans as 20% of calories and leaf vegetables as 10% of calories would contain 23% of calories as protein of high quality. An individual taking a diet containing 23% of calories as efficient protein would require an energy intake of only about 21 calories per kilogram, and since people taking grain-dominated diets normally have about 35 calories per kilogram available they should have no problem in meeting their protein needs with an SGA-type mix. An intake of 21 calories per kilogram amounts to only 1000 calories per day for a 105 pound woman and 1300 calories per day for a 135 pound man, which by Western standards is very low, but which proved to be completely adequate for adults taking primarily vegetarian diets in Ethiopia.[482]

If more than about 1300 calories were required by an individual taking the SGA basics additional calories could be derived from high-yield tubers and fruit since the 21 calories per kilogram of the wheat-bean-greens mix would cover requirements for protein and other nutrients.[483]

Mixes of plant proteins from legumes, leaves, grains and microorganisms have proven to be highly effective supplements to the diets of undernourished groups. Unfortunately, though, the mixes normally used are protein extracts or processed foods which are questionable nutritionally and inherently costly. It makes more sense to simply encourage those depending primarily on grains to plant more leaf vegetables, soybeans, legumes and tubers, especially potatoes (which have a very high yield per acre). It is not necessary to use precise amounts of specific foods to derive the benefits of mixing. It is only necessary to add a serving of soybeans or beans to the staple of the diet and take liberal amounts of raw leaf vegetables and potatoes.[484]

Adding vitamins and minerals to protein supplements is alleged to enhance their effectiveness, but the addition increases their cost and may introduce new problems. In the case of beans and other seeds, however, there is a safe, cost-free way in which to boost vitamin levels, namely by sprouting. Sprouting raises the already high vitamin levels of whole grains and beans threefold or more. Sprouting also tends to elevate protein content and to raise the availability of minerals. Moreover, sprouted seeds can, like greens, be eaten raw so that valuable vitamins are not lost in cooking. Cooking may adversely affect the availability of protein also.[485]

Studies have shown that pressure cooking and drying leaves meat protein essentially unusable. Heat may be even more destructive in the presence of sugars since reactions between certain sugars and amino acids result in substances the body can not utilize.[486]

New varieties of triticale, rice, corn and other grains containing high quality proteins may, as they become available, simplify the job of building better diets for the world's underfed. Large amounts of high quality protein may eventually come from algae, vegetable seeds, vines of vegetables and selected pulses. The Winged Bean which has been grown successfully on an experimental basis in Ghana, compares favorably nutritionally to soybeans and has a pleasant sweet taste in the raw state and should be even better sprouted.[487]

Attempts to improve the quality of proteins by supplementing them with purified amino acids have met with less than total success. Supplemental lysine failed to affect the growth of Indian children taking wheat-based diets, and failed to improve the utilization of wheat protein by Russian adults. In other studies it was noted lysine failed to raise the growth rates of rats taking rice, wheat, corn, soybean or millet, and children taking a grain-based diet responded better to the addition of leaf protein than to the addition of lysine to their diet. Supplementing the diets of preadolescent girls from low-income Southern families with methionine and other amino acids did not improve the efficiency of the protein in their diets. Supplementing the rice diets of Indian children with a mix of amino acids also failed to improve protein efficiency. While supplemental amino acids do enrich the pocketbooks of processors, they seem to do little for the people who use them. And what pure aminio acids do *to* people is simply not known.[488]

The food needs of the world's underfed can be met but factory foods are not the answer. Processing debilitates food nutritionally and wastes the limited resources of the poor nations. A step towards alleviating hunger would be increased production of greens, tubers, soybeans (or equivalent beans) and legumes, in addition to the utilization of used food sources, especially algae. The addition of such foods to grain-based diets would result in increases in quality and quantity of protein. And the high yields of tubers and greens would facilitate an increase in caloric intake which would serve to reduce total protein needs (and keep people from starving). Sprouting the legumes, soybeans and grains would raise protein levels still more and add richly to the amounts of available vitamins and minerals. The sprouting would also allow the whole diet to be eaten raw.[489]

PROTEIN DEFICIENCY IN THE U.S.?

Most of the work on protein deficiency has dealt with underfed nations, and Harvard's Dr. Mark Hegsted reported there is little evidence of protein deficiency in the U.S. Nevertheless ill-chosen diets could quite conceivably result in protein deficiency. Sugar, alcohol and fat contain no protein, and most fruits derive less than 5% of calories from protein. Processing reduces both the quality and quantity of protein of grains: cornstarch and corn oil, for example, contain no protein and the lysine content of wheat is cut about 30% in milling. Generally, then, products that have undergone a great deal of processing or cooking are suspect with respect to protein. And since there seems to be no bounds to dietary choices in the U.S. (ranging all the way from 100% alcohol or sweetened foods to almost total lack of carbohydrate) symptoms of protein deficiency may become buried beneath a myriad of other physiological and emotional problems.[490]

PART II: PROTEIN FOR GROWTH

Until now our discussion of dietary protein has dealt solely with maintenance requirements which constitute total needs for adults. Children share the need for protein for maintenance and require an additional amount of protein for growth since protein is the major constituent of new tissues. However, it is only during the first few months of life that protein requirements for growth exceed maintenance requirements so it is fortunate that we have a precise indicator of the magnitude of requirements during this critical period: human milk.[491]

Nutritionists of every denomination concede that human milk is perfect food for infants. In their classical textbook, *Nutrition*, Chaney and Ross point out that "advantages of human milk over cow's milk are well known" and they recommend babies be breast-fed for several months if possible. One of the few remaining defenders of animal fats, Dr. Roger Williams admitted that even modified cow's milk is inferior to mother's milk during early infancy. And Adelle Davis who staunchly supported high-protein diets, wrote "There is no question but that breast milk produced by a healthy mother is nutritionally far superior to any formula."[492]

What Adelle Davis failed to write is that mature human milk derives about 6.3% of total calories from protein whereas over 20% of the energy of cow's milk is derived from protein. Thus *cow's milk contains three times as much protein as human milk.*[493]

As a rule bottle-fed infants grow considerably more rapidly than those who are breast-fed. Cow's milk is not only much higher in protein but is on a par with human milk in fat content and high levels of fat serve to speed growth in their own way. Elevating caloric intake also boosts the rate of growth, and bottle-fed children normally have much higher caloric intakes than naturally fed children. Thus *cow's milk stimulates growth via high quantities of growth-promoting protein, high fat content and the ability to raise energy intake.*[494]

Actually there are many proteins that are on a par with cow's milk for stimulating growth. Backed by high fat and equal caloric levels many plant food mixes will match milk itself in promoting growth. A mix of chick peas, sesame flour and low-fat soy flour resulted in weight gains which matched those with cow's milk when fed to infants in the Middle East. The same was true of the highly touted vegetable protein mix, Icaprina. A mix consisting of cottonseed flour, bean flour and corn flour with a little yeast was equally effective in promoting the growth of children. After feeding a group of hospitalized 11- to 38-week-old infants a mix of chick peas, sesame flour and soybean flour, researchers concluded that the mix compared "quite favorably" with cow's milk. Malnourished Brazilian children experienced "nutritional recuperation" on a diet in which 60% of the protein came from a macaroni made from corn, defatted soy flour and wheat germ.[495]

Perhaps high intake of growth promoting protein and fat can aid in reversing the symptoms of undernutrition, but *low protein human milk is the preferred food for healthy infants.* The dangers of rapid growth and large body size have already been discussed. When rapid growth is carried beyond infancy, particularly when it results in increased body size, it leads to debilitating degenerative diseases. Dr. Mark Hegsted of Harvard estimates one-year-old infants require what amounts to about 5% of calories as protein which could be obtained from any whole-foods diet. The SGA diet should make a very good diet for weaning children. The idea of sprouting has been put to practice in a Pakistani mix called Camile II, which consists of sprouted wheat, beans and millet. Though SGA-type mixes have yet to be used by officialdom, green plants have been called "the largest unexploited source of protein" in the world. The protein of greens is high in the amino acid lysine, which restricts the utilization of grain proteins, (recall that supplementing the grain diet of a group of Indian children with leaf proteins, resulted in greater protein utilization than did the addition of lysine to their diet). Algae, which when added to sprouts and greens forms the basis for the SGA diet, constitutes still another untapped source of protein.[496]

The basic SGA diet derives about 20% of its total calories as protein, and if backed by sufficient caloric intake and fat the protein derived from the SGA diet would be highly effective in promoting growth. However, caloric requirements drop markedly with such a diet. The lower caloric intake would of itself reduce the tendency to promote growth, and as we have seen, maintenance needs, which constitute the bulk of protein requirements after the first few months of life, rise with a decreasing caloric intake. A 33% cut in calorie intake would more than double protein needs as a percent of calories. Requirements during weaning would thus reach over 10% of calories for a totally utilizable protein so that allowing for lack of complete digestibility and urinary losses the 20% level of the SGA diet does not look excessive. In any case the low calorie and low fat content of the SGA basics makes it certain the mix would not lead to excess growth. Adding easily digested vegetable foods such as baked potatoes, brown rice, fruits, etc., to the SGA basics would raise caloric intake and it would also lower protein as a percent of calories. The SGA diet should be suitable for children of every age since on the basis of percentage of calories, protein needs vary little from weaning through adolescence.[497]

Women should have no problem in meeting protein needs during lactation. The SGA diet would provide more than enough protein for milk production providing calorie intake were adequate. The same is true of pregnancy. Thus a sprout- green- seaweed mix, possibly supplemented by calorically rich foods, should make an excellent diet for the mothers of infants alike.[498]

6 / "fitness" diet vs. the SGA diet

The typical American diet is alarmingly low in a number of vital nutrients (see Appendix 4) and in the preceding chapters it has been shown that the U.S. diet contains pathological excesses of fat, salt, sugar, refined carbohydrates, cholesterol, calories, protein, purines, phosphorus, etc. In contrast to common American dietary items, sprouts and leaf vegetables are outstanding sources of virtually every known nutrient. The addition of a little seaweed to a mix of sprouts and greens forms the basis for the SGA diet which is complete with respect to nutritional needs and free from excesses. For comparison, we will use a diet based not on the average U.S. intakes, but on the recommendations of U.S. Department of Agriculture (USDA).[499]

Leaflet 424, Revised 1964, of the USDA is entitled "Food for Fitness" and gives A Daily Food Guide based on the popular "four basic food groups," namely the milk group, meat group, vegetable and fruit group and the bread and cereal group. For adults, the Food Guide recommends two or more cups of milk; two or more servings from the meat group; four or more servings of fruits and vegetables to include a citrus fruit or other sources of vitamin C, a source of vitamin A and potatoes; and four or more servings of whole grain or "enriched or restored" grain products.[500]

To consummate their mealtime masterpiece, the USDA recommends "other foods as needed to complete meals and to provide additional food energy and other food values." To "complete meals" American style is, of course, to add fats (butter, mayonnaise, cooking oil, etc.), sugar (with cereal, in jams, in coffee and other drinks, in canned fruits and vegetables, in pastries, sweets, etc.) and salt (in or on everything not containing sugar). The fats and sugar provide "additional food energy" and since fats usually provide at least some vitamin E and linoleic acid, salt is composed of sodium and chlorine and is sometimes supplemented with iodine and sugar adds glucose to the blood, it can be (and usually is) argued these three items offer "other food values." Thus, adding fat, sugar and salt to the "basic four" is in keeping with USDA recommendations.[501]

Exhibit F1 gives a quantitative list of specific foods which are in keeping with the USDA Daily Food Guide. Five ounces of sugar and five tablespoons of fat (as butter and margarine) round out the "basic four" selections. Since the USDA titles its work "Food for Fitness," the resulting food mix will be called the "Fitness" diet.[502]

Exhibit F1

The Fitness Diet

Linoleic Acid		Weight (grams)	Protein (grams)	Fat (grams)	CHO (grams)	Calories	Vitamin E (mg)
	MEAT GROUP						
0.5	4 ozs beef steak, grilled	114	28.7	24.6	neg.	346	0.2
2.3	2 ozs bacon, fried	57	13.6	26.1	neg.	298	0.3
0.4	one egg, fried	40	5.6	7.8	neg.	96	0.2
	MILK GROUP						
0.5	2 cups milk	488	16.6	18.0	23.6	322	0.15
	FRUIT AND VEGETABLE GROUP						
0.3	1 med carrot	50	0.5	0.1	4.8	21	.05
0.3	1 med orange	180	1.8	0.4	22.0	89	0.04
0.3	1 potato	110	2.3	0.1	18.8	84	0.1
0.3	Lettuce and tomato	160	1.7	0.3	6.5	31	0.43
	BREAD AND CEREAL GROUP						
0.6	3 slices bread (enriched)	60	4.8	0.8	31.0	144	0.03
6.1	1 serving cornflakes (enriched)	28	1.9	0.2	4.8	104	0.03
0.0	5 ozs sugar	142	0.0	0.0	141.0	547	0.0
.6	2 Tablespoons butter	28	0.0	28.0	0.0	250	0.28
1.8	2 Tablespoons margarine	28	0.0	28.0	0.0	250	3.8
1.0	1 Tablespoon mayonnaise	15	Trace	12.0	0.0	110	2.0
9.5	TOTAL	1500	77.5	146.4	252.5	2692	7.61

Exhibit F2 gives the particulars of a typical raw foods, sprout-green-algae (SGA) diet. It is shown to weigh under a pound and a half but this is based on dry weight of sprouts. As eaten, the SGA mix would weigh about four pounds compared to just over three pounds for the Fitness diet.[503]

Exhibit F2

The Sprout-Green plus Algae (SGA) Diet

FOOD	Weight (grams)	Calories (KCAL)	Protein (grams)	Fat (grams)	Linoleic Acid (grams)
Collards	150	67	7.2	1.2	.36
Turnip				
Greens	200	56	3.0	.3	.20
Parsley	50	22	3.6	.3	.10
Wheat				
Sprouts	200*	760	32.2	5.0	2.4
Mung				
Bean				
Sprouts	40*	125	13.6	.7	.36
Broad				
Bean				
Sprouts	20*	60	7.7	.3	.16
Soya				
Sprouts	60*	200	27.2	6.1	3.32
Lanenaria				
Saccharina				
(seaweed)	22	10	1.0	.2	.1
TOTALS	742	1300	95.5	14.4	7.00

*Dry Weight

CALORIES, PROTEIN AND FATS

The Fitness diet contains 2692 calories and 78 grams of protein. According to Exhibit P2 (*see Chapter 5*), this might lead to bone decalcification for any adult weighing under 143 pounds. And any increase in calories or protein would raise the risk of such a condition. The Fitness diet contains 146.4 grams of fat which represents 49% of total calories. This gross level of fat combined with a high protein and calorie level is the pathway to obesity, poor endurance and inactivity, psoriasis, shortened life expectancy, gout, kidney failure, various cancers and osteoporosis. High fat alone has been implicated in coronary heart disease, cancer, diabetes, multiple sclerosis, gallstones, arthritis, impaired hearing and strokes. Over 70% of the fat in the Fitness diet is derived from saturated animal sources which tend to elevate serum cholesterol and promote atherosclerosis. The presence of over 500 milligrams of cholesterol in the Fitness diet tends to further elevate serum cholesterol and raise the risk of cardiovascular disease, certain cancers, enlarged prostate glands and gallstones. Almost 90% of the cholesterol in the Fitness diet is derived from meat and eggs which are cooked before being eaten: heated cholesterol adds further to the risk of cancer. The animal fats in the Fitness diet are high in bile acids and oleic acid both of which have induced tumors in laboratory animals. Eggs and meat have been directly implicated in cancer, stone formations, psoriasis, obesity, heart attacks, strokes, osteoporosis and degeneration of the kidneys and liver.[504]

Aside from a small need for linoleic acid, humans are believed not to need any fat in their diet. A diet deriving 2% of the total calories from linoleic acid reportedly meets this need. Surprisingly the Fitness diet derives only 3% of total calories from linoleic acid. This does not mean, however, that cutting the fat level of this diet drastically would automatically create a deficiency of linoleic acid. Eliminating the beef, milk or butter from the Fitness diet would actually *raise* the fraction of calories provided by linoleic acid. Eliminating all of the animal products—beef, bacon, eggs, milk and butter—from the Fitness diet would reduce the fat content by 70% and still leave the linoleic acid level at 2.5% of calories. Presumably the USDA recommendations for meat and milk are based on the assumption that these products alone offer adequate amounts of protein. Indeed, eliminating the animal products from the fitness diet leaves a mix containing 1380 calories with only 13 grams of protein. But the vegetable products used (as part of the USDA plan) are anything but optimal.[505]

The totally vegetarian SGA diet contains 95 grams of protein with only 1300 calories—fewer calories, in fact, than the vegetable products alone in the Fitness diet. Moreover, the protein of the SGA diet is of highest quality. At first glance, the SGA diet might appear to contain an excess of protein but Exhibit P1 (*see Chapter 5*) shows this is not the case. As constructed the protein level of the SGA mix provides no more than minimal needs for adults weighing more than 121 pounds. Should individuals need additional calories they could take them as fruit, tubers, etc., thereby raising their total protein intake only slightly. Larger persons could add three or four tubers and a few hundred calories in fruits and vegetables to the SGA mix to satisfy their caloric needs. The additions would add about 10 grams of protein to the diet, but since total energy content would still be under 2000 calories (about 27 calories per kilogram for a 165 pound adult) there would still be no danger of an excess of protein.[506]

The SGA diet derives only about 10% of total calories from fat (compared to 49% for the Fitness diet) but half of this, or 5% of total calories, is derived from the essential linoleic acid (compared to 3% for the Fitness diet). The SGA regime contains no cholesterol, sugar or other refined carbohydrates, and it contains very little oleic acid and an insignificant amount of saturated fat. Evidently the SGA diet offers strong protection against the many disorders associated with fat-related substances.[507]

SUGAR

The USDA allowed the inclusion of five ounces of sugar (sucrose) and actually *recommended* refined grains in its Fitness regime. Through their role in producing hypoglycemia, sugar and refined grains have been implicated in irritability, mental depression, aggression, somnolence, insomnia and various forms of neurotic behavior. Sugar has been found to elevate serum lipids and triglycerides which raise the risk of atherosclerosis. Animals tend to incur fatty livers on diets high in refined carbohydrates, particularly sugar. Such build-ups may be aggravated by egg, which the USDA recommends and the Fitness diet dutifully offers. Refined carbohydrates and fat evidently work together in bringing on diabetes, and animal studies indicate sugar alone can cause the disease. Sugar and refined grains have been linked to cancer, obesity, arthritis, cataracts and smoking, and it is well known that sugar, like fat, alters the nature and amount of intestinal bacteria which tends to impair digestion and reduce the synthesis of essential nutrients. Sugar is known to be the most elemental cause of rampant tooth decay in the West. It causes the teeth of animals and humans to rot into dysfunctionality. Refined grains and sugar are neither necessary nor desirable additions to the diet.[508]

Plant foods contain varying amounts of natural sugars but even honey, which is almost all sucrose, does not match the action of pure sugar. There should be no danger in supplementing the basic SGA components with natural sugar-rich fruits. The basic SGA diet con-

tains about eight ounces of total carbohydrates, all of which are
contained in whole foods and very little of which are in the form of
sugars.[509]

VITAMINS AND MINERALS

The USDA's Fitness diet certainly seems to be a travesty in terms
of fat, protein, carbohydrate and related substances. On the other
hand, the strictly vegetarian SGA diet seems to be favorably disposed
with respect to these components. One would hope that the USDA's
recommendations would at least lead to adequate amounts of the
necessary minerals and vitamins. Exhibit F3 gives the amounts of the
various vitamins and minerals occurring in the Fitness diet. If the
levels of the B-vitamins in meat appear lower than those given in
some tables, it is simply that the losses due to cooking are taken into
account. Exhibit F4 gives the vitamin and mineral contents of the
foods in the SGA mix. It is assumed that all of the foods in the SGA
mix are taken raw. It would alter the vitamin levels only slightly
and the mineral levels none if the soybean sprouts were roasted. Judging by the experiences of those now enjoying the SGA diet, though,
the roasting is unnecessary.[510]

The total amount of each vitamin and mineral in the Fitness diet
and the SGA diet are summarized in Exhibit F5 which also gives the
minimum requirements for each nutrient based on available research
findings (*see Appendix 4*) and on the less inclusive Food and Nutrition Board Allowances.[511]

VITAMINS A AND C

The first thing that becomes clear from Exhibit F5 is that the Fitness diet contains adequate amounts of vitamins A and C. This is not
surprising since the USDA "Daily Food Guide," on which the Fitness
diet is based, specifies the inclusion of fruits or vegetables rich in A
and C. It might be surprising to some, then, that the SGA diet has
over four times as much vitamin A as the Fitness regime and more
than six times as much vitamin C. Green leafy vegetables are on a par
with carrots as a source of carotene and far outstrip oranges as a source
of vitamin C.[512]

The SGA diet contains no active vitamin D and the Fitness diet
little, but vitamin D is readily synthesized when the skin is given

direct exposure to the sun so there is no danger of deficiency for individuals who get plenty of sunshine. Thus unless the remainder of the diet reduces chances of getting sun exposure by rendering individuals inactive, vitamin D needs should represent no problem. Unfortunately, the high-fat, high-protein nature of the Fitness diet may, as noted earlier, tend to reduce activity levels. Lack of vitamin D could result in failure to absorb and utilize calcium.[513]

VITAMIN E

Vitamin E needs are above 0.3 milligrams per gram of fat, but the Fitness diet contains only a fifth of that amount. The SGA diet contains a high 1.2 milligrams per gram of fat and a safe 2.4 milligrams of Vitamin E per gram of linoleic acid. The SGA also satisfies the Food and Nutrition Board (FNB) recommendations with over 15 milligrams of vitamin E per day, but the Fitness diet offers only 7.6 milligrams of vitamin E. Thus the SGA contains an adequate amount of vitamin E based on any of three standards whereas the Fitness diet contains at best only a little over half the amount recommended. Vitamin E deficiency is not unlikely at the levels of the Fitness diet, especially since the amount of selenium in this diet is very low. Deficiency symptoms are varied but include the development of atherosclerosis and heart disease, slow wound healing, muscular dystrophy, infertility, liver and gland disorders and damage to the nervous system. The spinal cord and brain are affected by vitamin E deficiency in animals and saturated fat, in which the Fitness diet is extremely high, tends to increase the degree of paralysis resulting from vitamin E deficiency in laboratory animals.[514]

VITAMIN K

Little work has been done on the specific requirements for vitamin K, but from animal studies it appears needs are about 0.5 milligrams per day. The SGA diet contains over four times that amount of vitamin K, most of which is derived from green leafy vegetables, which are the only foods known to be rich in the vitamin. The Fitness diet apparently contains less than 20% of expected needs for vitamin K. The vitamin can, to a degree, be synthesized by bacteria in the intestines, but persons taking medicines and drugs or diets high in sugar and fat may obtain little or none of the vitamin from bacterial

Exhibit F3

Vitamins and Minerals in Fitness Diet

	BROILED BEEF STEAK 114 g	BACON FRIED 57 g	FRIED EGG 40 g	TWO CUPS MILK 488 g	ONE MEDIUM CARROT 50 g	ONE MEDIUM ORANGE 180 g	ONE MEDIUM POTATO 110 g	LETTUCE & TOMATO 160 g	THREE SLICES BREAD 60 g	ONE OZ. CORN-FLAKES 28 g	TOTAL
Vitamins											
A (IU)	51.0	0	456.0	600.0	5,500.0	360.0	Tr	1,460.0	Tr	0	8,427.0
C	0	0	0	9.0	4.0	75.0	22.0	30.0	Tr	0	140.0
D (IU)	0	0	35.0	5.0	0	0	0	0	0	0	40.0
E	.20	.30	.2	.15	.05	.04	.1	.43	.03	.03	1.53 [1]
K	<.01	<.01	.01	very low	low	low	low	fairly low	very low	very low	<.1 mg
Thiamin	0.07	0.19	0.03	0.15	.03	.2	.1	.1	.15	.12	1.14
Riboflavin	.15	.06	.14	.82	.025	.08	.04	.06	.12	.02	1.51
Niacin	4.0	1.3	.03	.49	.3	.2	1.6	.96	1.4	.6	10.8
Pyridoxine	.37	.18	.07	.19	.07	.11	.18	.14	.05	.02	1.38
Pantothenic Acid	.37	.20	.72	1.6	.14	.45	.4	.48	.18	.06	4.6
Biotin	.002	.003	.006	.023	.0012	.0006	.0001	.006	.002	.002	.046
Folacin	.003	.001	.001	.0029	.004	.004	.008	.005	.009	.0015	.039
B_{12}	.0011	.0004	.00008	.0019	some	some	0	0	Tr	0	.0035
B_{17}	low	low	low	low	some	some	some	some	low	low	poor
P	Low	Low	Low	Low	some	high in peel	some	some	low	low	very poor w/o orange peel
R (grain)	.0	.0	.0	.0	.5	.2	.55	.8	.12	.2	2.37
U					some	some	some	little			low

Minerals

											[2]
Ca	10.0	30.0	25.0	585.0	10.0	74.0	8.0	32.0	52.0	3.0	829.0
P	345.0	136.0	104.0	464.0	14.0	36.0	58.0	43.0	48.0	17.0	1,265.0
Na	76.0	1,760.0	88.0	244.0	2.0	2.0	3.0	6.0	310.0	290.0	2,781.0
Cl	73.0	2,710.0	79.0	480.0	13.0	5.0	100.0	80.0	395.0	430.0	4,365.0
K	420.0	264.0	70.0	780.0	125.0	360.0	450.0	400.0	66.0	32.0	2,967.0
S	306.0	170.0	83.0	140.0	4.0	19.0	25.0	13.0	47.0	26.0	833.0
Mg	29.0	14.0	6.0	68.0	7.0	20.0	24.0	21.0	14.0	5.0	208.0
Fe	5.9	1.8	1.0	.4	.5	.7	.7	1.6	1.1	.8	14.5
Zn	1.7	1.1	.5	1.7	.12	.30	.5	.40	.6	.5	7.4
Mn	.006	.016	.016	.1	.15	.06	.44	.48	.24	.06	1.57
Cu	.10	.24	.07	.1	.04	.4	.19	.13	.11	.05	1.43
I		.009	.005	.02	.001		.004	.003		.001	.043
Se	.032	.01	.005	.007	.001	.002	.001	.0016	.01	.001	.07
Mo	.008	.16	.02	.1			.003	.05	.02	.05	.4
Cr	.01	.006	.006	.005			0.	.005	.003	.001	.036
V	low	low	low	low	low	low			low	low	low
F	low	low	low		low				low	low	tends to be low
Linoleic Acid (grains)	.5	2.3	.4	.5	.3	.3	.3	.3	.6	.6	6.1
Ash pH (milli-equivalents)	26.0 acid	5.0 acid	6.0 acid	tends to be acidic	3.0 basic	8.7 basic	5.5 basic	6.2 basic	1.8 acid	.7 acid	16.1 mg acid

[1] Fats raise vitamin C content to 7.61 milligrams.
[2] Fats raise linoleic acid content to 9.5 grams.

Exhibit F4

Vitamins and Minerals in Basics of a Particular SGA Mix
(in milligrams unless specified otherwise)

	COLLARDS 150g	TURNIP GREENS 200g	PARSLEY 50g	WHEAT SPROUTS 200g (dry wt)	SOY SPROUTS 60g (dry wt)	MUNG SPROUTS 40g (dry wt)	BROAD BEAN SPROUTS 20g (dry wt)	SEAWEED 22g	TOTAL 742g
Vitamins									
A(IU)	13,900.	15,200.	4,200.	300.	300.	700.	40.	500.	35,140.
C	228.	278.	86.	80.	57.	68.	64.	8.	869.
D(IU)	0.	0.	0.	0.	0.	0.	0.	little	little
E	3.0	4.0	.9	2.6	6.0	.7	.3	—	17.5
K	.75	1.0	.25	.1est	.05est	.04est	.02est	.04	2.2
Thiamin	.24	.42	.06	1.8	1.01	.46	.17	—	4.20
Riboflavin	.46	.78	.13	1.04	.98	.46	.38	—	4.23
Niacin	2.5	1.6	.6	20.6	3.5	2.8	2.0	—	33.6
Pyridoxine	.23	.20	.10	1.4	.36	.44	.10	—	2.83
Pantothenic Acid	.45	.76	.015	5.10	1.0	1.0	.24	—	8.57
Biotin	.005	.006	.0002	.072	.036	.003	.002	—	.124
Folacin (free)	.105	.084	.02	.08	.09	.048	.088	—	.515
B_{12}	—	—	trace	small amt.	small amt.	some	—	.003	.003
B_{13}	some	roots rich	some	apparently high	apparently high	unknown	unknown	—	more than adequate

B_{15}	some	roots rich	some	apparently high	apparently high	unknown	unknown	—	more than adequate
B_{17}	fair source	fair source	fair source	good source	good source	best known source	good source	—	very high
R (grams)	1.8	1.6	.75	5.2	3.5	2.5	.4	.5	16.2
P	excellent source	excellent source	excellent source	good source	good source	good source	good source		very high
U	excellent source	excellent source	excellent source	good source	good source	good source	good source		very high
Minerals									
Ca	375.	492.	101.	54.	210.	68.	18.	—	1,318.
P	123.	116.	32.	700.	300.	200.	150.	—	1,621.
Na	65.	88.	22.	6.	90.	30.	50.	144.	495.
K	300.	300.	75.	625.	1,000.	1,200.	450.	220.	4,170.
Mg	85.	116.	21.	282.	175.	120.	37.	—	836.
Fe	.12	3.6	3.1	7.2	8.2	4.5	3.6	3.5	36.0
Zn	—	7.0	—	10.8	1.2	—	.6	1.4	>21.0
Mn	3.0	3.8	.6	8.4	1.7	.6	.3	.2	18.6
Cu	12.	.16	.26	1.2	.66	.3	.29	—	2.99
I	—	—	—	—	—	—	—	10.	10.
Se	.008	.010	.0025	.13	.01	.006	.003	—	.17
Mo	.07	.09	.03	.10	.37	.26	.08	—	1.0
Cr	.006	.008	.002	.03	.006	.004	.002	—	.058
F	.01	.01	.005	.01	.3	.005	.002	>.5	>.84

EXHIBIT F5

Estimated Requirements for Vitamins and Minerals and the Amounts in the Fitness Diet and the SGA Diet

(Values given on per day basis unless otherwise specified)

(in milligrams unless otherwise specified)

VITAMIN	APPROXIMATE MINIMUM DAILY NEED FOR ADULT HUMANS	FITNESS DIET	SGA DIET	FNB/NAS–NRC RDDA—revised 1973	
				ADULT MALE	PREGNANCY
A	4000 IU (6000 IU in pregnancy	8400 IU	35,146 IU	5000 IU	5000 IU
C	90 (115 in pregnancy)	140	869	45	60
D	None with adequate sun exposure, otherwise about 100 IU	35 IU	small amt.	400 IU	800 IU
E	.3 mg/g animal fat .9 mg/g vegetable oil or 1.7 mg/g linoleic acid	7.6 mg total .06 mg/g fat 1.2 mg/g linoleic acid	17.5 total 1.2 mg/g vegetable oil 2.4 mg/g linoleic acid	15	15
K	0.5–2.0	<.1	2.2		
Thiamin	>.4 mg/1000 cal. and >.7 mg	0.41 mg/1000 cal.	3.2 mg/1000 cal. (4.2 total)	1.4 (.5 mg/1000 cal.)	1.7 (.65/1000 cal.)
Riboflavin	.6 mg/1000 cal. .8 mg/1000 cal in pregnancy	.55 mg/1000 cal.	3.2 mg/1000 cal. (4.23 total)	1.6 (.6 mg/1000 cal.)	1.9 (.87/1000 cal.)

Niacin	>4.4 mg/1000 cal. and >8.8 mg	3.9 mg/1000 cal.	25.5 mg/1000 cal. (33.6 total)	18 (6.7 mg/1000 cal.) 18 (8.5 mg/1000 cal.)
Pantothenic Acid	3 mg/1000 cal.	1.66 mg/1000 cal.	6.6 mg/1000 cal. (8.6 total)	
Biotin	50 μg/1000 cal.	20 μg/1000 cal.	100 μg/1000 cal.	
Pyridoxine	30 μg/g protein	18 μg/g protein	30 μg/g protein (2.8 total)	2.0 2.5
Folacin	100 μg (free) (150 μg free in pregnancy)	39 μg (free)	515 μg (free)	400 μg (total) 600 μg (total)
Cobalamin	.3 μg (.5 μg in pregnancy)	3.5 μg	3.0 μg	3.0 μg 4.0 μg
B_{17}	Unknown	Very low	Outstanding	
P	Unknown	Very low	Outstanding	
U	Unknown	Very low	Outstanding	
B_{13}	Unknown	Probably low	More than adequate	
B_{15}	Unknown	Probably low	Probably high	
R (grams)	7 g/1000 cal. and >10 g total	.85 g/1000 cal. 2.4 g total	13 g/1000 cal. 16.2 g total	
Lineolic Acid	>2% Calories	2.7% Calories	5.0% Calories	
Fat	<15% Calories	40% Calories	<11% Calories	

continued →

Exhibit F5 (continued)

(1) 2780 mg Na without iodized salt and 3240 mg with 1g iodized salt
(2) 1.07 without iodized salt and .85 with 1g iodized salt
(3) 43 μg without iodized salt and 130 μg with iodized salt
(4) Based on dry wt. of sprouts, wet wt. of greens

MINERAL	APPROXIMATE MINIMUM DAILY NEED FOR ADULT HUMANS	FITNESS DIET	SGA DIET	FNB/NAS-NC RDDA—revised 1973
Ca	400–500	829	1118	800
Ca:P (ratio)	.67 or more	.78	.67	1.0
Na	Preferably under 1000	(1)	495	
K:Na (ratio)	Over 1.5	(2)	over 8.0	
I μg	About 100	(3)	10,000	130
Mg	300–400	208	836	350
Zn	8	7.4	over 21.0	15
Fe	5–10 men; 10–20 women, 30 during pregnancy	14.5	36.0	10 men; 18 women
Cu	1.5–2.0	1.43	2.99	
Mo	About .6	0.4	1.0	
Mn	3–5	1.57	18.6	
Se	.1–.3 ppm (.0033–.01 mg/1000 cal.)	.04 ppm .0022/1000 cal.	.25 ppm (4) .013/1000 cal.	
Cr	up to .1 if sugar intake high	.04 (and high in sugar)	>.05 with no sugar	
V	Probably about .1 particularly important if fat intake high	probably low (and high in fat)	Probably high	
F	Probably about .1 particularly important if sugar intake high	high	Adequate	
Acid-Base Equiv.	Optimum 10–30 meq basic	16.1 meq acid	22 meq basic	

synthesis. It is not surprising to find evidence that vitamin K deficiency is common in the U.S., especially among middle-aged and elderly persons. Deficiency is associated with hemorrhaging and failure of the blood to coagulate which results in vulnerability to internal bleeding, accidents, operations, childbirth, etc.[515]

THIAMIN, RIBOFLAVIN AND NIACIN

Thiamin requirements are put at something in excess of .4 milligrams per 1000 calories which amounts to more than 1.1 milligrams for the 2692 calorie Fitness diet. The Fitness diet contains 1.1 milligrams thiamin which probably would prevent deficiency symptoms under normal conditions but might elicit problems during pregnancy. The SGA diet contains a remarkable 3.2 milligrams of thiamin per 1000 calories and more than double the FNB recommendation for pregnant women in spite of the fact the diet contains only 1300 calories. If the Fitness diet does prove to be low in thiamin, it is likely to lead to damage to the central nervous system, resulting in irritability, depression and confusion.[516]

Vegetarian diets are not always high in riboflavin, but the SGA diet abounds with 3.2 milligrams riboflavin per 1000 calories and over 4 milligrams total. Needs are of the order of 0.6 milligrams per 1000 calories and under 2 milligrams total. The Fitness diet falls slightly short of this with a content of 0.55 milligrams per 1000 calories and its total of 1.5 milligrams riboflavin is 20% below the FNB recommendations for pregnant women. The high fat content of the Fitness diet might, in the presence of the marginal levels of riboflavin, lead to nervous disorders.[517]

The Fitness diet contains about 3.9 milligrams niacin per 1000 calories and a total of 10.9 milligrams niacin. Minimum needs total about 4.4 milligrams per 1000 calories and the FNB suggests an intake of 18 milligrams per day. The deficit would be more than made up by the conversion of the amino acid tryptophan to niacin if the pyridoxine level of the fitness diet were adequate, but the pyridoxine content of the Fitness diet is exceedingly low. Thus, there is at least some possibility that the Fitness diet may lead to niacin deficiency symptoms. Nervous disorders including loss of memory, hallucinations and depression could result. The SGA diet contains about 26 milligrams niacin per 1000 calories which is almost six times the minimum requirements. This is augmented by a high level of tryptophan and a supply of pyridoxine which is adequate to support conversion of tryptophan to niacin.[518]

The Fitness diet contains enriched bread and refined cereals which are supplemented with niacin, riboflavin and thiamin. The niacin and riboflavin levels in the Fitness diet are further enhanced by the fact that the two vitamins are considerably more resistant to cooking than other water soluble vitamins. It would thus be expected that the amounts of niacin, riboflavin and thiamin in the Fitness diet would be relatively high. However, the Fitness regime proved to be, at best, marginal in these popular vitamins. By way of contrast, the supplement-free SGA diet provides five to seven times the estimated minimum requirements for niacin, riboflavin and thiamin. The contrast between the two diets is even more striking with respect to some of the lesser known, but no less important, water soluble vitamins.[519]

PANTOTHENIC ACID

A pantothenic acid intake of 3 milligrams per 1000 calories appears to be adequate whereas the Fitness diet contains only 1.7 milligrams per 1000 calories which could result in declining levels of the all-important coenzyme A. The SGA diet provides a rich 6.6 milligrams pantothenic acid per 1000 calories. As with the other vitamins involved in carbohydrate metabolism, deficiency of pantothenic acid tends to effect neurological changes. A shortage of the vitamin may lead to irritability, insomnia, somnolence, fatigue, headaches, cramps, restlessness and gastrointestinal changes. Purveyors of pills for these common disorders are not likely to be ardent supporters of the SGA diet.[520]

BIOTIN

Closely related to pantothenic acid, metabolically, is biotin. Recommended intake of biotin is about 50 micrograms per 1000 calories. The SGA diet contains about two times that amount, but the Fitness diet offers less than half of the recommended 500 micrograms per 1000 calories. Biotin can be synthesized by the intestinal flora but, sucrose (table sugar) and lactose (milk sugar), in which the Fitness diet are high, tend to prevent adequate synthesis in animals and presumably act in a similar fashion in man. Drugs and high fat levels may also impede intestinal synthesis. In man, biotin deficiency may bring on increases in serum cholesterol and nervous disorders in the form of lassitude, somnolence and depression.[521]

VITAMIN B$_6$

Needs for pyridoxine (Vitamin B6) depend to a large extent on the level of protein in the diet. When protein intake is excessive, as may be the case with the Fitness diet, B6 needs mount rapidly. When protein is not excessive, B6 needs should be covered by an intake of 20 micrograms of B6 per gram of protein but with an excess of protein in the diet, B6 needs increase by 50% or more. Thus the Fitness diet which contains an excess of protein and less than 20 micrograms of B6 per gram of protein tends to be very low in the vitamin. The SGA diet contains more than 30 micrograms B6 per gram of protein which should be more than adequate since the diet does not carry an excess of protein. The basic SGA diet contains 2.8 milligrams of pyridoxine total, which is above the FNB recommendation of 2.0 milligrams for normal adults and 2.5 milligrams during pregnancy.[522]

The total B6 content of the Fitness diet is some 25% under the FNB recommendation for normal adults and 40% under the FNB quota during pregnancy. Lack of B6 may result in hypoglycemia (low blood sugar), disturbed glucose tolerance, fatty liver, nervous disorders, kidney stones, atherosclerosis, tooth decay, inadequate production of antibodies, mental illness and convulsive seizures. Pregnant women and infants are particularly vulnerable, and athletes may require a high level of the vitamin. They are certainly not going to receive it with the USDA's Fitness diet.[523]

FOLACIN

Normal adults need an estimated 100 micrograms of free folacin per day and pregnant women need up to 150 micrograms per day. The SGA offers over 500% of normal needs and over 300% of needs during pregnancy. On the other hand the Fitness diet provides only 39% of normal needs and 26% of needs during pregnancy. Heavy cooking losses, losses during refining and the choice of foods which are not good sources of folacin account for the anemic level of folacin in the Fitness Diet. Deficiency is associated with macrocytic anemia, severe reduction in antibody formation, cancer and toxemia during pregnancy. The Fitness diet must be regarded as grossly low in folacin particularly for pregnant women and anyone under stress.[524]

VITAMIN B$_{12}$

Adults evidently require less than .5 micrograms of dietary vitamin B$_{12}$ per day. There is no evidence of B$_{12}$ deficiency among East Indians taking as little as .16 micrograms of B$_{12}$ per day. In spite of this, the FNB recommends 3.0 micrograms of B$_{12}$ per day for normal adults and 4.0 micrograms of B$_{12}$ per day during pregnancy. The Fitness diet provides 3.5 micrograms of B$_{12}$, while the SGA diet contains 3.0 micrograms of the vitamin. Both levels are probably more than ten times minimal needs.[525]

VITAMIN P

No specific requirement for vitamin P has been established, but the Fitness diet is low in the vitamin. The only good source of vitamin P in the Fitness diet is the peel of the orange, which the FNB does not recommend eating and which the public invariably discards. The sprouts and greens in the SGA diet are all rich in vitamin P. A good supply increases muscular capacity and endurance and may enhance vitamin C utilization. Deficiency may lead to edema, degeneration of capillary walls, kidney disorders and impaired carbohydrate metabolism.[526]

VITAMIN B$_{17}$

The Fitness diet is very low in the anticancer nitrilosides, or vitamin B$_{17}$. The SGA is rich in B$_{17}$ since sprouts are the richest source of the vitamin. There is evidence that B$_{17}$ not only protects against the onset of cancer, but is effective in treating existing tumors. The fat, calories, protein, heated cholesterol, lack of roughage, sugar, refined grains and shortage of numerous nutrients in the Fitness diet all raise the risk of cancer, but the diet offers little in the way of defense from nitrilosides. There appears to be no chance of contracting cancer with the SGA diet, but if malignant cells were to appear there is a good supply of B$_{17}$ to deal with them.[527]

VITAMIN B$_{15}$

Pangamic acid, or vitamin B$_{15}$, reportedly occurs in some of the same foods in which vitamin B_{17} is present. Presumably, then, the SGA diet contains an adequate and possibly rich supply of B_{15} but the Fitness diet may be low in the vitamin. Vitamin B_{15} has been effective in treating a variety of conditions including heart disease, eye disorders and pneumonia; pangamic acid evidently plays a role in fat metabolism and may serve to protect the liver. Working with vitamin P, pangamic acid may facilitate an increase in the liver supply of glycogen and keep serum cholesterol down. Deficiency of pangamic acid may render the body more susceptible to a variety of disorders related to lipid metabolism and reduce the body's capacity to repair itself and recover from injury.[528]

VITAMIN U

The cabbage family, which includes greens, is the principle source of vitamin U, the antiulcer vitamin. Other fresh vegetables contain the vitamin also. Thus, the SGA diet provides a large amount of vitamin U, whereas the meager array of vegetables in the Fitness diet would be expected to provide little of the vitamin. A low level of vitamin U may lead to gastritis and gastric ulcers.[529]

VITAMIN R

Proper movement of food constituents and waste products through the intestines requires up to 10 grams of roughage (vitamin R) depending on body size. The Fitness diet contains only 2.4 grams vitamin R, but the SGA diet contains over 16 grams of the vitamin. The effects of R deficiency may include much more than incessant constipation, discomfort and intestinal degeneration associated with diverticulosis. Coronary heart disease, various cancers, appendicitis and other major degenerative diseases are believed to be related to deficiency of this oft-overlooked nutrient. Epidemographical studies show those who take whole-foods, more vegetarian diets, hence high levels of vitamin R, suffer far less from the major degenerative diseases than those eating more refined, more animalistic diets like the Fitness regime.[530]

VITAMIN B_{13}

The milk in the Fitness diet should provide some orotic acid (vitamin B_{13}). The greens in the SGA diet are good sources of B_{13}, and the level could be boosted substantially by eating the turnips with the turnip greens. Deficiency of B_{13} is associated with liver disorders and disturbances in carbohydrate metabolism. The high levels of sugar, fat and cholesterol in the Fitness diet pose a severe threat to the liver, and are quite likely to result in impaired carbohydrate metabolism. Thus the need for B_{13} is apt to be greatly elevated for anyone taking the Fitness diet. A deficiency could result.[531]

The vitamin tally shows the Fitness diet with three clear adequacies (vitamins A, C and B_{12}), four marginal cases (thiamin, riboflavin, niacin and orotic acid) and 11 inadequacies (vitamins E, K, B_6, B_{17}, P, U, B_{15} and R, plus pantothenic acid, biotin and folacin). This assumes exposure to the sun is sufficient to effect synthesis of an adequate amount of vitamin D. With adequate sun exposure, the SGA diet offers an adequate amount of every vitamin listed and most levels are high multiples of needs.[532]

There is no simple way to eliminate the vitamin shortages in the Fitness diet. Substituting whole wheat bread for enriched white bread would boost vitamin R some 40%, but pyridoxine, pantothenic acid, folacin and vitamin E levels would be increased only 5% to 12% whereas increases of 50% to 200% are called for. The switch would not improve biotin levels and would effect decreases in riboflavin and thiamin.[533]

Doubling the meat content of the Fitness diet would do little or nothing for the vitamin shortages and would aggravate problems associated with high levels of fat, protein, calories, cholesterol, etc. Adding an egg to the Fitness regime would elevate the level of pantothenic acid but still leave the diet far short of estimated needs. And the extra egg would do little for other shortages while boosting heated cholesterol levels markedly.[534]

Doubling the milk in the fitness diet to a quart per day would lessen the severity of the deficits of pyridoxine, pantothenic acid and biotin and shore up riboflavin levels. But no deficiencies would be expected to disappear and the fat-bloated fitness diet would become even higher in its excesses of saturated and total fat, cholesterol, protein and lactose. A calorie-for-calorie substitution of milk for flesh (beef, bacon and eggs) would lower the niacin content but it would raise the level of pantothenic acid, riboflavin and biotin. The switch would reduce total protein, hence make more pyridoxine available to aid in converting tryptophan to niacin. *Thus abandoning the first of the "four basic food groups," namely, the meat group, should lead to an across-the-board improvement in vitamin levels.* Fat content would be reduced also. The change might bring on some problems with mineral levels, particularly copper, however.[535]

Substituting beans or soybeans, rather than milk, for the flesh in the Fitness diet would be a far greater boon to vitamin levels; sprouting the beans and taking the sprouts raw would effect a striking increase in the vitamins levels. But this should come as no surprise, since it would make the Fitness diet look more like the SGA diet. Substituting greens like the ones in the SGA diet for the milk and/or vegetables in the Fitness diet would shore up levels of vitamin A, C, E, K, B_{15}, B_{17}, P, U and R, along with riboflavin, niacin, pyridoxine, pantothenic acid, folacin and possibly orotic acid. Vitamin B_{12} levels would go down, but the reduction could be more than offset by combining the greens with sprouts and the peanut-like flavored sweet-tasting seaweed, laminaria saccharina, that the Scots call "sugar wrack."[536]

Evidently the more the USDA's Fitness diet is altered to take on the appearance of the SGA diet, the stronger it becomes. But the picture is not complete without an examination of mineral levels in the two diets.[537]

CALCIUM

The mineral which probably receives the greatest amount of publicity is calcium. With a low-fat, whole-foods diet, which is commensurately low in calories and protein, the requirement for calcium is probably less than 400 milligrams per day, provided phosphorus content is not excessive (*see Appendix 4*). The FNB recommends 800 milligrams of calcium per day and both the Fitness diet, with 829 milligrams, and the SGA diet, with 1318 milligrams cover this.[538]

The normal calcium-phosphorus (Ca:P) ratio of the U.S. diet is about 1:3 and with such an excess of phosphorus any level of calcium might prove to be inadequate. Surprisingly, the Fitness diet has a more favorable calcium-phosphorus ratio of 1:1.5, but if one were to raise the amount of meat, eggs and grain products in the USDA's

Fitness diet to normal levels, the ratio would be far less favorable. The SGA diet also has a Ca:P ratio of 1:1.5.[539]

SODIUM, POTASSIUM AND IODINE

Concern over sodium intake is usually centered on how to avoid an excess rather than how to get enough. Low-sodium diets have been used to treat high blood pressure, hyperthyroidism, kidney disorders, heart disease, edema and other maladies. "Salt-free" diets are the basis for almost all "nature cures"; Drs. Max Gerson, Henry Bieler, C. Leslie Thomson and the renowned hygienist Herbert Shelton all regard salt as a major health hazard. The Fitness diet contains 2.8 grams of sodium which is some ten times actual needs. Sodium intakes exceeding 1.0 grams per day are suspect. The SGA diet, with 0.5 grams of sodium is more than adequate.[540]

The risk of high sodium intake is reduced by a high level of potassium in the diet and potassium deficiency can result from a low ratio of potassium to sodium (K:Na). The K:Na ratio should exceed 1.5:1 but the Fitness diet has a ratio of only 1:1. The SGA diet maintains a very favorable K:Na ratio of more than 8:1.[541]

The basic Fitness diet contains only 40 to 50 micrograms of iodine, which could lead to a hypothyroid condition and goiter. Minimum needs for iodine total about 100 micrograms per day, and the FNB recommends about 130 micrograms per day. The normal way Americans shore up their iodine intake is to include iodized salt in the diet. One gram of iodized salt would lift the iodine level of the Fitness above 100 micrograms, but the price of this is an elevation of sodium intake and a further reduction in the K:Na ratio. With one gram of iodized salt, the K:Na ratio would drop from an already low 1.0 to .85 and with normal salt levels the ratio would fall by about 70%. An alternative to the iodized salt would be a small amount of dried seaweed. A mere gram of "sugar wrack" would provide over 300 micrograms iodine and add less than .03 grams sodium to the diet. The minute amount of seaweed improves the K:Na ratio also since seaweeds have K:Na ratios above 1.0. Ten grams of dried sugar wrack would raise the sodium content of the Fitness diet only 10% and provide .6 to 1.2 milligrams of vitamin B_{12} so that the high sodium products in the diet—meat, eggs and milk—could be eliminated completely: sprouts and greens would cover the needs for all other necessary nutrients.[542]

The changes would of course transform the Fitness diet into something fit to be called a diet, that is the SGA diet, which contains about 10,000 micrograms iodine. Raw greens and high iodine intake tend to reduce absorption of iodine, suggesting the extraordinary amount of iodine in the SGA diet is not as high in relation to needs as it first appears. But there should be no danger from iodine deficiency with the SGA diet: goiter is almost unknown in Japan where seaweed is a common foodstuff. At the same time, there is no reason to classify the iodine content of the SGA diet excessive since persons with normal thyroids do not react adversely to high iodine intake.[543]

MAGNESIUM

In Appendix 4 it is shown that minimum needs for magnesium total at least 300 to 400 milligrams per day for men and over 250 milligrams per day for women. And it is quite possible that magnesium needs are considerably above these levels. The SGA diet contains over 800 milligrams of magnesium which is safe by any standards, but the Fitness diet contains only about 200 milligrams of magnesium which is low by any standards. The FNB calls for 350 milligrams of the mineral. The Fitness diet's magnesium content would be elevated by 25% by simply substituting whole wheat bread for "enriched" white bread. Doubling the amount of bread in the diet and substituting whole wheat bread for white bread would push magnesium levels up to 300 milligrams per day. This would, of course, require reducing intake of some other items to keep calorie intake from going even higher. Candidates for elimination include beef, bacon, eggs, sugar, margarine, mayonnaise and butter. The low level of magnesium in the Fitness diet could lead to impaired carbohydrate metabolism and emotional disorders. Symptoms of deficiency include irritability, excitability, depression and personality changes. Physiological symptoms include intestinal disorders, kidney afflictions, including stone formation, bone degeneration and cancer.[544]

ZINC

Under ideal conditions, adult needs for zinc are probably on the order of 8 milligrams per day. However, high protein, calcium, calories, sugar and phytic acid intakes tend to raise the need for zinc which may explain why the FNB recommends an intake of 15 milligrams per day. The SGA diet contains over 21 milligrams of zinc, including about 15 milligrams of the mineral free from phytic acid and soy protein (which may tend to render zinc unavailable). The Fitness diet contains only 7.4 milligrams zinc, about 6 milligrams of which is free from phytic acid. Thus the Fitness diet has no margin of safety to protect against its high calcium, protein, sugar and calorie levels. It is doubtful the Fitness diet would lead to deficiency symptoms but the possibility can not be disregarded: levels are at best marginal. Deficiency might result in lethargy and rough skin.[545]

IRON, COPPER AND MOLYBDENUM

Iron needs are on the order of 10 milligrams per day for men, 20 milligrams per day for menstruating women and 30 milligrams per day for pregnant women. The FNB recommends 10 milligrams per day for men, 18 milligrams per day for women and says the increased requirement during pregnancy "cannot be met by ordinary diets." But the extraordinary SGA diet contains 36 milligrams of iron, without the addition of foods to meet increased calorie requirements, which would boost iron levels even more. The Fitness diet contains 14.5 milligrams of iron, and women, who require up to 20milligrams iron per day, would normally take fewer than the 2692 calories in the Fitness mix which could bring their iron intakes down to a very low 13 milligrams or less per day.[546]

Most of the iron in the Fitness diet is derived from meat and eggs, but substituting mung bean sprouts for the flesh products on a calorie-for-calorie basis would more than double the iron content. Replacing the milk with 14 ounces of greens would be still another way of doubling the iron content. Replacing an ounce of any item in the Fitness diet with an ounce of seaweed would boost iron levels over 20%. Thus any path to making the Fitness diet look more like the SGA regime will lead to stronger iron levels.[547]

Without some changes the Fitness diet would leave many women, particularly pregnant ones, in danger of iron deficiency anemia. Pregnant women taking 15 milligrams of iron per day or less were found to have low hemoglobin levels, and two thirds of a group of college women were found to have scant supplies of iron.[548]

Requirements for copper are thought to be about 1.5 to 2.0 milligrams per day. Copper is believed to be necessary for the absorption of iron so a low copper level may aggravate a deficiency in iron. The iron-poor Fitness diet contains only 1.4 milligrams copper which could but increase the risk of iron deficiency. The iron-rich SGA diet contains a high 3.0 milligrams of copper. Replacing some of the milk in the Fitness diet with parsley would represent an improvement in both iron and copper levels as would replacing the flesh foods with bean sprouts. Earlier it was indicated that substituting milk for flesh foods in the Fitness diet might adversely affect copper levels. Milk is a very poor source of copper. Milk diets are used to induce copper deficiency in animals and have been implicated in copper deficiency in children. Lacto-vegetarian diets (as the Fitness diet would be with milk replacing flesh which includes eggs) tend to be low in available copper unless they include a substantial amount of sprouted beans, onions or certain greens, including parsley. Severe copper deficiency might not only result in anemia but could lead to damage to the pancreas, brain and reproductive system.[549]

Although copper aids iron absorption it tends to leave iron in a state in which iron can not be used in the production of red blood cells. Molybdenum, on the other hand, is believed to play a role in preparing iron for use in red blood cell production. The Fitness diet provides about 380 micrograms molybdenum whereas some 600 micrograms are believed to be needed for adequate production of red cells. The SGA diet contains about 1000 micrograms molybdenum. A high copper-molybdenum (Cu:Mo) ratio tends to aggravate low molybdenum intake, and the Fitness diet has a Cu:Mo ratio of over 4:1 whereas the SGA diet has a ratio of 3:1 which is recommended. Low molybdenum serum levels are common in iron deficiency anemia, and molybdenum deficiency may result in more than just anemia. Lack of the mineral may lead to kidney stones, particularly when the diet contains a high level of flesh products. Gastrointestinal disturbances and diarrhea may also be involved. The most direct path to correcting the anemic level of molybdenum in the Fitness diet is to use bean sprouts to replace flesh foods, fats or sugar.[550]

MANGANESE

Kindergarten-aged children require about 5 milligrams of manganese per day and 5 milligrams per day was found to be adequate for adults. Presumably, though, adults' needs are little, if any, less than 5 milligrams per day. The SGA diet includes a high 18.6 milligrams of manganese whereas the Fitness diet contains a mere 1.57 milligrams of the mineral. Manganese deficiency may be involved in such common conditions as poor lactation and birth defects; bone deformities and calculus result from low intake by animals.[551]

CHROMIUM

The exact requirement for dietary chromium is not known, but it is known that refined cereals, fats and oils and sugar contain little of the mineral. The high level of these items in the U.S. diet has left Americans with a much lower intake of chromium than individuals elsewhere. There is every reason to believe the Fitness diet is no higher in chromium than the normal American regime. But the SGA diet, which contains no degradants or extracts and is high in whole grains and beans, should be extremely rich in chromium. Chromium is associated with glucose tolerance, and the low level of chromium in the Fitness diet might, in time, lead to diabetes. The low level of chromium in the U.S. diets is suspected of playing a role in rising incidence of diabetes with age.[552]

SELENIUM

The need for selenium has been estimated to be at least 3.3 milligrams per 1000 calories. The SGA diet provides an abundant 12.7 milligrams per 1000 calories, but the Fitness diet contains only 2.2 milligrams per 1000 calories. The low level of selenium in the Fitness diet raises further the risk of vitamin E deficiency. As noted earlier, the Fitness diet is very low in vitamin E and selenium tends to have a sparring effect on vitamin E. In addition to symptoms of vitamin E deficiency, the lack of selenium in the Fitness diet might lead to damage to the pancreas and the reproductive organs.[553]

FLOURINE

The addition of 0.7 to 1.0 ppm fluorine to drinking water is alleged to provide a measure of protection against dental decay, but water supplies containing more than 2 ppm tend to result in mottled enamel. The sprouts and greens in the SGA diet contain an estimated .6 ppm fluorine, and seaweed, which is believed to be the richest food in fluorine, should boost this to .7 ppm or more. Individuals who take the SGA diet rarely drink liquid: the diet contains little sodium and over three pints of water in foodstuffs so individuals seldom have any need or desire for water or any other liquid. Using fluorinated water in sprouting would boost the fluorine content of the SGA diet but the addition could lead to an excess of fluorine. The high level of salt in the Fitness diet is certain to cause a need for additional water so that fluorine would be picked up by anyone taking the Fitness diet and relying on fluorinated water for drinking purposes. It is sheer fantasy to envision a lifetime of freedom from tooth decay with the Fitness diet, however. There is overwhelming evidence that sugar, refined grains and lack of a host of vitamins and minerals cause dental decay. After decades of fluoridation, dentists' businesses continue to grow and a billion caries now stand in need of treatment in the U.S. alone.[554]

OTHER MINERALS

Vanadium, boron and several other elements may, in time, achieve recognition as necessary micronutrients. Vanadium, for example, may play roles in preventing tooth decay and keeping serum cholesterol levels down. Beans, soybeans, whole grains and other whole seeds contain relatively large amounts of a broad spectrum of possible micronutrients. But refining takes a heavy toll, suggesting a diet like the Fitness regime is likely to be low in such minerals. The SGA diet contains a large quantity of mineral-rich, whole seeds and a measure of seaweed which is far and away the most concentrated food source of minerals. The SGA mix is strengthened further by leaf vegetables which stand out among vegetables as a mineral source.[555]

MINERAL ASH

The pH of the blood remains in a very narrow range of 7.32 to 7.47 and is thus basic in nature. A drop of pH below 7.3 is manifest acidosis while a rise above 7.55 reflects alkalosis. Either condition threatens the survival of body cells and both conditions are uncommon. But the price of prevention can be high when the diet is acidic.

Calcium is a vital buffering agent, and highly acidic diets lead to bone resorption and reductions in skeletal integrity. It has been shown that the normal U.S. diet leads to substantial losses in bone density during middle age and beyond. High-protein and/or high-meat diets cause rapid losses of bone density in even young adults. The U.S. diet is high in sulfur, phosphorus and chlorine, which are acid forming, and contains not enough base-forming potassium, sodium, calcium and magnesium to buffer the acid forming minerals. Clearly any diet which is at all acidic will require buffering action after it is absorbed. Thus a slightly basic diet, probably in the range of 10 to 30 milliequivalents basic, should be optimal. Without the seaweed, which is high in chlorine, hence acidic, the SGA diet would be highly alkaline; as structured it offers a favorable 22 milliequivalents base balance. The Fitness diet, on the other hand, is acidic to the extent of 16 milliequivalents acid. The latter could, and evidently would, lead to debilitating bone resorption.[556]

MINERAL SCORE CARD

Now let's take an overall look at minerals in the two diets. The mineral tally shows the Fitness diet with five adequacies (calcium, phosphorus, iodine, iron and fluorine), eight probable deficiencies (potassium, magnesium, zinc, copper, molybdenum, manganese, selenium and chromium) and one excess (sodium) for men taking iodized salt. For women taking iodized salt, iron deficiency must also be regarded as probable, and the reading is four adequacies, nine deficiencies and one excess. The same reading holds for men not taking iodized salt. Women not taking supplementary iodine would face ten deficiencies, three adequacies and one excess. Capping this disturbing array of deficiencies is an acidic ash from the minerals is the Fitness diet.[557]

The SGA diet has an abundant supply of every mineral for which there is believed to be a need. It contains rich surpluses of iodine, calcium, iron, magnesium, manganese, zinc, copper, molybdenum and potassium. It offers favorable ratios of calcium-phosphorus, iron-copper, potassium-sodium and copper-molybdenum. The bulk of every one of the minerals in the SGA diet is readily available: the greens are comparatively low in oxalates, the soybean and bean sprouts are ridded of most of their phytates and impediments to absorption. Factors that adversely affect utilization such as cooking, high fat intake, imbalances and processing are not present. The pH in the SGA diet is mildly basic, as in the blood.[558]

THE AGGREGATE

On an aggregate basis, the Fitness diet maintains acceptable amounts of no more than 11 vitamins and minerals; at least four of these are marginal and two more depend on supplementation. It contains low levels of 19 to 21 vitamins and minerals and carries an excess of sodium. It appears to have an adequate amount of linoleic acid, but it carries excesses of oleic acid, purines, total fat, saturated fat, total cholesterol, heated cholesterol and possibly protein. It contains a gross excess of sugar, and refined cereals and protein-calorie levels are undoubtedly excessive for many individuals. Thus the Fitness diet is buried in at least 11 excesses, all of which depend on the presence of animal products, salt and refining. Dietary excesses tend to elevate the needs for vitamins and minerals but the Fitness diet, with 20-odd deficiencies, is unfit to meet even normal needs. The final stigma on this diet based on "the four basic food groups" is an acid ash which can lead to degradation of the skeletal structure, if not deterioration of the internal environment in the form of acidosis.[559]

Can a diet recommended by the U.S. government be so poor? Is not the USDA's "Food for Fitness" a step above the average? If so, why are there no reports of deficiency diseases or conditions resulting from dietary excess? Or are there?[560]

To deal with the last question first, let us examine the probable consequences of deficiencies of the nutrients which the Fitness diet appears inadequate and the expected consequences of the alleged excesses. Exhibit F6 lists the likely deficiencies and the most probable result of deficiency of the nutrient. Exhibit F7 lists the alleged excesses and the most likely response to such excesses. None of the conditions resulting from these deficiencies and excesses are unavoidable but all are common, if not universal, in America today. Heading the list are emotional disorders, including irritability, depression, restlessness, lassitude, somnolence, insomnia, fatigue and insanity. Heart disease, strokes, diabetes, high blood pressure, atherosclerosis and degradation of blood vessels are related to a number of deficiencies and excesses in the Fitness diet. Cancer is related to at least seven of the overages and deficiencies. Aspects of the Fitness diet have been implicated in obesity, anemia, kidney and gall stones, brain damage, pneumonia, poor eyesight, aging, early mortality and multiple sclerosis. Other imbalances are believed to be related to appendicitis, ulcers, intestinal disorders, constipation, diarrhea, acidosis and gastric disturbances. Headaches, tooth decay and even smoking may result from diets like the Fitness diet. It is doubtful that anyone eating the typical American diet, or its not-so-well-masked representative in the form of the USDA's "Food for Fitness" regime, can live a full life, free from the afflictions listed in Exhibits F6 and F7.[561]

Exhibit F6

Likely deficiencies associated with the U.S.D.A.'s Fitness diet and symptoms of said deficiencies.

LIKELY DEFICIENCY	PROBABLE SYMPTOMS
Vitamin E	Atherosclerosis and coronary heart disease; strokes; muscular dystrophy; infertility
Vitamin K	Hemorrhaging
Pantothenic Acid	Irritability, insomnia, somnolence, fatigue, headaches, restlessness
Biotin	High serum cholesterol, lassitude, depression
Pyridoxine (vitamin B_6)	Low blood sugar, poor glucose tolerance, kidney stones, fatty liver, tooth decay, poor resistance to disease, insanity
Folacin	Anemia, poor resistance to disease, cancer, toxemia during pregnancy
Vitamin P	Degradation of blood vessels, kidney disorders, diabetes
Vitamin B_{17}	Cancer
Vitamin B_{15}	Pneumonia, poor eyesight, fatty livers
Vitamin U	Ulcers, gastritis
Vitamin R	Constipation, coronary heart disease, appendicitis, cancer, diverticulosis
Potassium	High blood pressure
Iodine (without supplement)	Goiter
Magnesium	Excitability, irritability, depression, personality changes, kidney stones, intestinal disorders, cancer
Zinc	Lethargy, rough skin
Iron (without supplement)	Anemia

Exhibit F6 (continued)

LIKELY DEFICIENCY	PROBABLE SYMPTOMS
Copper	Injury to brain, pancreas and reproductive organs, anemia
Molybdenum	Kidney stones, diarrhea, anemia
Manganese	Birth defects, poor lactation
Chromium	Diabetes
Selenium	Pancreatic conditions, all symptoms of vitamin E deficiency

Exhibit F7

Apparent excesses in U.S.D.A.'s Fitness diet and probable consequences of excesses of said substances.

SUBSTANCE	PROBABLE CONSEQUENCES OF EXCESS
Fat	Obesity, coronary heart disease, strokes, atherosclerosis, diabetes, multiple sclerosis, cancer, gall bladder stones, poor endurance, aging, high serum lipids, arthritis
Saturated Fat	Atherosclerosis, coronary heart disease, strokes, high serum cholesterol, high serum triglycerides
Cholesterol	High serum cholesterol, atherosclerosis
Heated cholesterol	Cancer
Oleic Acid	Cancer
Purines	Gout, stone formation
Calorie-Protein	Obesity, osteoporosis (bone degeneration), cancer, shortened life expectancy, degenerative diseases
Sodium-Chlorine	High blood pressure, hyperthyroidism
Sugar-Refined Carbohydrates	Tooth decay, depression, aggression, lethargy, smoking, objectionable body odor, cancer, coronary heart disease, low serum glucose, disturbed glucose tolerance, insanity, multiple sclerosis, shortened life expectancy, criminality
Phosphorus-Chlorine Sulfur (acid ash)	Acidosis, loss of bone calcium and magnesium, aging

But others, including the Hunzas and Abkhasians do, and the diets of the Hunzas and Abkhasians are not as rich and balanced nutritionally as the SGA diet. Although the Abkhasian diet bears little resemblance to the Fitness diet, it does include processed grasses, in the form of dairy products, vis-à-vis fresh raw greens; the Hunza diet includes cooked beans and grains in lieu of raw, sprouted ones (though the Hunzas do take some sprouts). And both diets lack mineral- and vitamin B_{12}-rich algae.[562]

Minor changes in the Fitness diet improve the levels of certain nutrients, but they leave the diet with many vital shortages. Replacing the enriched bread with whole wheat bread would elevate manganese levels to a marginal status and raise magnesium levels from about 50% of needs to over 60% of needs. The substitution would strengthen low copper and zinc levels and narrow the wide gaps between intake and needs for vitamin E and R. Combining a switch to whole wheat bread with a doubling of the amount of bread in the Fitness diet might eliminate four deficiencies, but deficiencies would still outnumber adequacies and excesses would go unabetted. Replacing flesh with dairy products would aggravate a shortage of copper unless the change was accompanied by a doubling of bread intake and a switch to whole wheat bread. A far more effective path to shoring up nutrient levels would be to replace meat with bean sprouts but the latter move would simply be a step in the direction of replacing the Fitness diet with the SGA regime.[563]

With sun exposure so that an adequate amount of vitamin D is provided, the SGA diet would make available rich, but not excessive, amounts of every vitamin and mineral for which there is evident need. It would also provide substantial amounts of minerals and possibly other nutrients whose need may yet be established. It has a favorable basic ash and tolerably low levels of sodium and chlorine.[564]

The SGA diet contains only one tenth as much fat as the Fitness diet, and yet is on a par with the Fitness diet in the amount of linoleic acid which is the only necessary fatty acid. It contains no cholesterol, heated or unheated, a very low level of oleic acid, no bile components and less saturated fat than a single bite of beef. It is low in purines and offers an adequate, but not highly excessive, level of good quality protein with a minimum of calories.[565]

The U.S. Government evidently puts the financial interests of the ranchers, feed lot operators, slaughter houses, meat packers, wholesalers, dairy cattlemen, milk processors, milling giants, agribusinessmen, supermarket chains, bankers, chemical companies, confectioneries, bottlers, paper companies, etc. above the health of the people. Their "four basic food groups" are four brutal farces. Their "fitness" diet is fit for no one who is truly health conscious, as we all should be. A mushrooming segment of Americans are in effect saying "no thank you" by turning to simplicity, the essence of which is vegetarianism, the ultimate of which may be the SGA diet.[566]

7 / survival

ORGANIC FARMING

It is gratifying to watch the revival of organic farming in the U.S. and Europe. Attempts to accelerate natural growth patterns through the use of chemicals have resulted in illusory gains in yields and have effected a marked decline in quality. Organically grown foods tend to be nutritionally superior, and individuals who avoid salt, oil, cooking and other agents that mask and destroy the taste of foods, find organically grown foods are far tastier. Naturally grown foods are spared contamination by a host of harmful chemical residues, and organic methods enhance the quality of the soil. Chemical-dependent farming jeopardizes long term productivity by disrupting local ecosystems and threatens our reeling biosphere by leaving in its wake death-oriented insecticides, herbicides and fungicides.[567]

Unfortunately, not all organic farming is clean farming, environmentally. When practiced on a scale of large acreage, organic farms require heavy, sophisticated farm machinery for plowing, tilling, planting, crop protection and harvesting. Special structures and irrigation systems may be involved, and storage, processing and transport to distant market places is usually required. Equipment requires iron and other metals, plastics, rubber, fabrics, etc., which not only deplete dwindling supplies of metal ores and petrochemicals but require large expenditures of energy for their extraction, processing and fabrication. Once in use, machinery and equipment require constant maintenance and intermittent overhauls. At every stage of production and use, machinery drains dwindling supplies of raw materials and with every expenditure of a resource, pollutants enter the biosphere.[568]

ECOLOGICAL FARMING

An alternative to the brand of organic farming which pollutes and draws heavily on natural resources is self-reliance on small plots, or ecological farming. Ecological farming need not lead to so-called subsistance, but if it is to supply the farmer and his family with their food and fiber needs, it certainly must lean towards reliance on plant foods, i.e. provide a primarily, if not totally, vegetarian diet.[569]

The reasons those engaged in ecological farming must rely on plant foods can be made clearer by a specific example. South-central Texas receives an average annual rainfall of about 40 inches, and though the area is warmer than most of North America, its soil is not overly productive. However, some corn (maize) is grown in the area and in 1973, average yields totaled 42 bushels or about 2500 pounds of corn per acre. Soybean yields were about 20 bushels or some 1200 pounds per acre. Corn is normally planted in mid to late March and harvested in late August or early September. Soybeans are planted in late May and harvested during October and November. Green leaf vegetables can be planted before and after the soybean harvest and collected throughout the winter, spring and early summer. Yields of green leaf vegetables would be expected to exceed 15,000 pounds per acre per year. Another high-yield crop is potatoes which can be planted in February and collected after soybean planting. Yields for potatoes average about 15,000 pounds per acre in the area. Conveniently the timing of the planting and harvesting of the four crops namely corn, soybeans, greens and potatoes spreads the work load out over the whole year so there is little pressure to seek the aid of machinery and equipment to relieve peak work loads.[570]

An adult's yearly food needs could be met with one and a half bushels of corn and a bushel of soybeans for sprouting plus 550 pounds of green vegetables and 1100 pounds of potatoes. On the basis of 1973 production figures in south-central Texas, this would require 0.036 acres of corn, 0.05 acres of soybeans, .0365 acres of greens and .073 acres of potatoes. The total is just under a fifth of one acre so that a family of four could, if they obtained average yields, get by on 4/5 of an acre of harvested land. However, these figures are deceptive since they reflect the results of intensive farming techniques. Intensive farming is associated with the use of chemical fertilizers and hybrid varieties which are efficient users of these chemicals, a procedure which threatens the delicate balance of life supporting minerals in the soil. Intensive farming requires life-taking chemicals aimed at dealing with insects, weeds and viruses, but which result in ever more resistant varieties of weeds and insects, destroying the life substance of soil and threatening the well-being of their users with increasingly potent residues. Intensive methods call for a degree of mechanization which sanity forbids.[571]

If our hypothetical south-central Texas family of four decided to avoid being caught up in the need for large scale operations to pay for resource-depleting, biosphere-polluting chemicals and equipment, they might find their yields were considerably lower than average, at least initially. A hundred years ago corn yields were only half of what they are today in the U.S. Some of the gains could be obtained by choosing hybrids which increase yields without demanding intensive fertilizing, by fertilizing with composted vegetable and animal wastes and rock salts, by making use of natural antagonists to insects and weeds and by taking advantage of the wind for powering irrigation pumps. Additional gains could be expected from the personal care "gardening" implies. But the net result is apt to be lower than average yields, especially during the critical early years. If we assume output would be two thirds the average, our four south-central Texans would need about 1.2 acres of harvested land. If the land were to be left idle every third year, they would need about 1.8 acres of tillable land or a total land area, including a house lot and small plot for additional vegetables, some fruits and a little cotton, of about 2½ acres. The actual amount of land planted and harvested each year would be about 1¼ acres (a shade less than the area of a football playing field, including the end-zones). By double-cropping total acreage could be reduced, of course, and families settling in more productive areas would require considerably less cropland. Based on average U.S. yields, adjusted to reflect the absence of chemical inputs, a total land area of about 1½ acres should suffice for a family of four. This amounts to about a third of an acre per person.[572]

U.S. TODAY

Since modern farmers use so many "aids" to boost output it might be expected that less than a quarter acre of cropland per person would be necessary to supply the U.S. with food. Actually there is about ten times this much, or 2.5 acres per person devoted to cropland. In addition to the cropland, there is about 2.5 acres of animal grazing land per person so that some five acres of farmland is being used to feed one average American. The U.S. actually has 3.5 to 4 acres of land suitable for cultivation per person. Using ecologically sound organic methods, the nation should be able to supply the food needs of 60% of the world's current population. The U.S. is currently feeding less than 7% of the world's inhabitants.[573]

Only half of the cultivatable land in the U.S. is actually producing crops and only 20% of the crops produced are used for human food. Most of the harvested acreage goes to feeding animals, and up to one acre of potential cropland per person is being used for grazing. Grazing animals currently occupy about half the land suitable for cropland plus almost half of all of the remaining land.[574]

Over a billion people could be fed with only the land used for animals in the U.S. Two thirds of the world is going hungry simply because Americans choose to eat meat and other animal products. Animal products account for most of the money spent on U.S. farm products, but these products account for only a third of total calories consumed. Ironically eliminating animal products from the diet of North Americans should cause no increase in the need for plant foods since the basal metabolism is lowered substantially when meat is eliminated from the diet. Meat-eating is always expensive calorically. The essentially vegetarian Hunzas, who enjoy a winter of Arctic proportions, take less than half as many calories as the meat-eating Eskimos. The caloric intake of the Hunzas is less than 60% that of Americans, and the de facto vegetarian Ethiopians who live in a warm climate take far fewer calories than even the Hunzas.[575]

CRUX OF THE PROBLEM

The reason it takes such an enormous amount of land and resources to meet America's demand for animal products is again the fact that the conversion of plant foods (feeds) to flesh and dairy products is very inefficient. It takes 11 pounds of corn to put one pound on a steer, and only about half the steer's carcass is used for meat so it takes about 22 pounds of corn to produce a pound of meat. Moreover, the pound of meat contains a third fewer calories than a pound of corn so it takes over 33 pounds of corn to produce the caloric equivalent of a pound of corn as beef. Putting land into tubers yields about 50 times as much food energy as would be derived from meat.[576]

Normally when authors and reporters call attention to the inefficiency of meat-eating, they base their comparison on available protein. A pound of meat protein requires about ten pounds of corn protein, but this is a poor comparison for when land is devoted to say tubers and greens, it yields up to 50 times as many calories as when the land is used for animal feeds, and when an individual derives adequate energy from tubers and leaf vegetables he obtains an abundant supply of protein. You may recall from the discussion of protein that virtually any whole food contains more than enough protein in relation to calories. On the other hand, a high protein intake does not lower calorie needs. In fact meat tends to boost caloric needs.[577]

Perhaps the reason so much utter nonsense is accepted as basic truth about protein is that the acceptance benefits almost everyone financially albeit no one physically, morally or spiritually. We equate "good" times with times of full employment. We equate "good" jobs with high-paying jobs. And we equate the "good" life with doing nothing which is what dead people do.[578]

To show how including meat in the diet affects one's lifestyle, and indeed forces upon us the gross excesses of our way of life, let us consider again our family of four in south-central Texas. With an all plant-food diet, they would need about 2½ acres of total land. Let us suppose that they decide to include a half pound of beef in the daily diet of each member of the family. In order to corn-feed enough steers to produce 730 pounds of beef a year, the family would need to produce an additional 16,000 pounds of corn or an additional ten acres of harvested corn. With five acres for crop rotation and 2½ for the cattle to live on, total land needs would go up to 20 acres or eight times the 2.5 acres needed with a vegetarian diet plan. Plowing, tilling, etc., almost 12 acres each year would require some form of mechanization. Horses or mules might be used but their food needs would push crop needs still higher. If we assume five acres would suffice for the beasts of burden, the total land requirements would be raised to 25 acres or ten times the requirements with the vegetarian diet. Initial investment and maintenance needs would be expanded markedly with the need for fences, water, grain storage, feed bins, gang plows, a seeder, harrow, wagons, etc., not to mention the animals themselves. Cash crops or some other source of revenue would be required to pay for and maintain the facilities. To obtain a gross income of just

$2,500 per year from corn would require more than doubling the scale of the farm. But such an expansion makes the use of a tractor look much more attractive, if not necessary. The implications in terms of additional needs for land, capital and income pressure one to seek avenues to more efficient production techniques. An "idealistic" family might decide to forego chemical sprays and fertilizers, but this would only raise further the demand for resource-depleting, energy-consuming and costly machinery and implements.[579]

The decision to eat meat makes simple self-sufficient farming impossible. Indeed the demand for animal products is the very foundation of large scale, mechanized farming in the U.S. With a vastly superior vegetarian diet, the nation's food needs could be met by the use of 5% of its land area; at present over 50% of the nation's land is set aside for farming. But it would be economical foolishness and moral debauchery to idle most of the United States' cultivatable land when so much of the world needs food. Particularly when the world's needs could be met by farming in ways which require a minimum of natural resources and which improve soil, air, water and quality of food produced.[580]

The motivation for switching to an SGA-type diet in primarily vegetarian countries like India may be stronger than the motivation for the change in the meat-eating nations. In India, as in most of Latin America and Asia and much of Africa, diets tend to be dominated by a single cooked grain. Sprouting these grains and taking the sprouts raw would raise vitamin levels at least threefold; it would enhance the availability of minerals, it would elevate protein content and it would all but eliminate motivation for refining and the use of salt, oil and spicy condiments. The production of soybeans and legumes for sprouting would give rise to still further improvements in the traditional grain-based diets. However, the biggest boon to such diets is apt to be the addition of large quantities of fresh, raw dark green, leaf vegetables which would boost intake of vitamins A, U, K, E, P, B_6, B_{13}, B_{17} and C plus riboflavin, folacin, pyridoxine, biotin and pantothenic acid. The eating of leaf vegetables would also bring about big increases in dietary calcium, iron, manganese, magnesium and other minerals. Deficiencies of a number of these nutrients play an important part in the vulnerability to disease of children taking cooked grain diets or the milk of mothers taking such diets. There is no question, though, that lack of an adequate amount of food is an important part of the problem. To alleviate this basic problem, India and other countries could turn to greater use of tubers, especially potatoes, as well as green vegetables. The amount of calories derived from land devoted to greens and tubers is substantially greater than the calories derived for land used for grains and legumes which in turn is far greater than the calories derived from animals fed the grains and legumes.[581]

Although it requires a degree of repetition, it will be instructive to compare the land requirements for various diets in the grain-eating areas. To this end, let us use figures for India where there is currently less than an acre of arable land per person.[582]

Based on Indian production figures it would require over five acres of land to supply the food needs of a single individual eating the normal U.S. diet. It may be recalled that it actually requires about five acres of farmland per person to supply the U.S. with its food. Yields tend to be lower in India than in the U.S., but based on Indian production estimates, the food needs of an individual taking the SGA diet could be met with a quarter of one acre of land.[583]

Thus, *the normal U.S. diet requires twenty times as much land as the SGA diet*. These staggering differences in land requirements are the result of three factors. First is the fact that it takes about 22 pounds of feed grain to produce a pound of meat. Second is the fact that the amount of food energy derived from an acre of greens, fruit or tubers in India is several times the food energy derived from an acre of grain: about 80% of the calories of the SGA diet are derived from tubers, greens and fruit while only about 20% comes from sprouts. Third and last is the fact the caloric requirements for individuals taking the SGA diet are 20% to 50% less than for individuals taking the normal U.S. diet.[584]

It should be clear that an Indian setting out to provide a meat-rich diet for himself, much less for his family, would be in trouble without the use of machinery and equipment. Anyone who has done a little gardening knows a 20′ x 30′ plot can occupy a lot of time. The five acres necessary to supply a single person with a meat-based diet constitutes over 350 such plots, and the acreage necessary to supply a small family with a meat-based diet would entail in excess of 1000 such plots land-wise. Ecological (and logical) farming is vegetarian farming.[585]

Of course the use of five acres of farmland per person in India is out of the question. There are only two acres of total land per person in India, and for all practical purposes land for food must be kept under a half acre per person. As noted the SGA diet would facilitate production of an individual's food needs on only a quarter acre (and without the use of intensive farming techniques). However, a grain-based diet requires over a half acre of land per person and leaves India in a situation in which food output is low and getting worse as population mounts. *The SGA diet would apparently allow India to feed double its current population.*[586]

Ignoring the advantages of green vegetables and tubers, Western "experts" continue to advocate the use of special high-yield grain varieties which often require irrigation and always require intensive use of chemical fertilizers, insecticides and herbicides. Even with the use of these costly inputs, the amount of food produced falls short of what the output would be if the same amount of land were used to organically grow tubers and greens. Also the application of chemicals would threaten the health of the soil, water, air and inhabitants of the area, especially those who eat the treated grains. As previously stated the supply of chemicals depends on vanishing world supplies of petrochemicals and minerals, and it requires cash expenditures which could be diverted to purchases of needed foodstuffs. In a back-handed way, technologists acknowledge the advantages of green leaf vegetables by recommending the use of leaf protein extracts of the greens. The use of leaf proteins and chemical-dependent grain varieties may fatten the profits of chemical companies, oil producers, food processors, machinery makers, shippers, etc., but it offers only promises to the people of India as well as others in Asia, Africa and Latin America.[587]

It might be argued that a change in diet could only be a stop-gap measure in alleviating the problem of overpopulation. Indeed a change to better diets would speed growth rates unless birth rates declined. On the other hand, lowering the average number of children born to two per family would of necessity stabilize world population regardless of how much life expectancy were increased. Families tend to be large where marriages take place at very young ages and child mortality rates are high. To find examples of population groups where the number of children rarely exceeds two per family we need only to turn to the same three groups so often cited in this book for their joyful miens, longer years of life and unusually good health: namely the Abkhasians, Hunzas and Vilcabambas. The Abkhasians rarely have more than two children and it is traditional with the Abkhasians to wait until their 30's to get married. This, of course, seems absurd to Westerners who, because of their animal-rich diets, mature very young and who by their 30's, are "over the hill." Getting married after age 30 is equally out of place in areas where individuals must fend for themselves by their early teens. On the other hand, the practice of marrying at later ages is not unique to the Abkhasians (whose youth are now beginning to abandon the ways of the past). The simple-eating ancient Maya formed matrimonial bonds at even later ages.[588]

The age at which the Hunzas and Vilcabambas marry, and the number of children they have is important. Both groups, especially the Hunzas, take even less animal protein than the Abkhasians and, the Hunzas' diet is closer to the SGA diet than the diet of any known group. While exact averages of the number of children per family do not seem to be available for the two groups, neither group is marked by large families. And in spite of their excellent health which prevents childhood deaths as well as promoting long life, neither group is large. Vilcabambas are very small and, in spite of a long history, there are only about 50,000 Hunzas. And unlike the Abkhasians, of whom there are over 100,000, the Hunzas were not periodically attacked and reduced in numbers by outsiders. Thus, there is reason to believe a good diet is entirely compatible with, if not the primary reason for, control of population.[589]

In closing it is fitting to enumerate some of the possible consequences of the adaptation of a diet based on sprouts and greens, vis-à-vis meat and sugar, in the U.S.[590]

The health of the population should improve dramatically. Degenerative disease—cancer, coronary heart disease, strokes, diabetes, hypertension, atherosclerosis, colds, hearing and vision defects, dental caries, diverticulosis, calculus (stones), obesity, etc., should all but disappear. The discontent, isolation, anxiety and lethargy that infest society would be expected to yield to active, involved attitudes and behavior. Life span should, in time, be at least doubled with the elderly remaining alert, strong and durable with perfect teeth, eyesight and hearing.[591]

The economic consequences of true health go far beyond eliminating the need for dentists, medical practitioners, drugs, hospitals, pharmaceuticals, medical equipment and so forth. For example, the elimination of circulatory disorders should allow people to enjoy greater environmental extremes. As a result designers might in many cases forego central heating and air conditioning and take advantage of such factors as the heat storage capacity of thick clay walls and the "breathing" capacity of straw.[592]

Vibrant health would no doubt bring a surge in activity levels and a desire to get about on foot or on bicycles. If accompanied by an interlocking system of public transportation and cycling paths, autos could become a thing of the past.[593]

Most of the world may eventually find itself hard pressed to supply its food needs even with an SGA type of diet. They could probably supply their own vegetables, but more and more they may have to turn to the land-rich nations for grains and legumes. As potential suppliers of grains and legumes for up to six billion people, the U.S. could expect unprecedented trade surpluses. Only a handful of nation can reach its potential as a food supplier if it channels its crops into feed for animals. The Soviet Union, for example, produces enough grain to feed its own people plus all of Africa and Europe. But a growing demand for meat has induced the Russians to feed their own grain and imported soybeans to animals, and as a consequence, they have had to import U.S. wheat to feed their own people.[594]

Economists may question the ability of densely-populated, energy-poor nations to pay for food imports. One way this might be done is through labor intensive production of quality goods. If one craftsman from each family relying on U.S. grains gave up only 15% of his output for U.S. grains each year then every man, woman and child in the U.S. would be able to enjoy the production of two months labor of a full-time skilled craftsman from the exchange.[595]

The production of grains for export could be accomplished by the continued use of chemical fertilizers, pesticides and the like, but a shift to plant foods would no doubt lead to severe cutbacks in the use of artificials. A concerned public would certainly demand an end to the polluting effects of farm chemicals, and the profit-oriented defenders of chemicals could no longer argue that chemicals were necessary to keep food prices down and to assure our food supply. Scientists estimate that eliminating fertilizers without a change in the diet would raise food prices only about 11%, and it is likely food prices would actually decline with production outstripping U.S. needs some tenfold. Never should it be forgotten that the true costs of intensive farming must include penalties for the lower quality and pollution associated with farm chemicals (as should the costs of meat and sugar include the damage to the body and mind).[596]

The scale of production, i.e. average size of farm, would be expected to drop markedly as more persons sought the independence of self-sufficiency. It would benefit society to encourage a trek to small farms; cities would be spared the stifling growth of recent decades; the soil, air and water would be improved, the food supply would be improved; and with a need for vast numbers of farmers the U.S. would be spared massive unemployment so that the era of "economic growth" would come to an orderly, rather than violent and catastrophic, end.[597]

This century and especially the post-World War II period is earmarked by an ever increasing output of industrial goods. An astounding array of mass-produced items has caused North Americans to produce their own weight in refuse in a matter of days and induced Africans and Asians to put their meager accumulations of cash into transistorized radios, soft drinks and ball-point pens. The lifestyle associated with the age of consumption has two sides: it puts the user of goods and gadgets in the position of a king with a court of mechanical, electrical and electronic slaves, but it has been accompanied by deteriorating mental and physical health, inactivity, fear, violence and a paradoxical trend toward isolation and dependence on others. Overlooked in the past was the environmental impact of uninhibited quest for industry's offerings. And so accustomed to more are those in industrialized societies that "need" for new automobiles takes precedence over the "luxury" of unpolluted air.[598]

TOMORROW

If sanity has lost its hold, reality has not. The "oil crisis" of 1973 was the first tremor of what promises to be the end. With the growth in the use of petroleum following the trend set since 1900 the known reserves will be depleted within 25 years. This will mean an end to not only the world's most versatile fuel source, but a drying up of the primary source of raw materials for plastics and other petrochemical products.[599]

While much verbiage has been given to the oil situation, the insatiable industrial complex threatens to deplete the world of all of the minerals of which "man-made" goods are actually made. The Interior Department reports an industrialized society depends on 13 basic raw materials. Four of these, namely copper, lead, zinc and tin are headed for depletion before the world's oil runs out. Though not classified as basic, the available supplies of gold, silver, molybdenum, mercury and platinum are expected to be used up in the next two decades. If iron output were to grow no faster than the 3.8% per year seen during the 60's, we could expect reserves to last about 70 years. It has been the practice, however, to alloy much of the iron with manganese, nickel and tungsten, the availabilities of which are expected to end long before iron ore reserves are depleted. The supply of galvanized iron promises to wane in the next ten to 15 years as known zinc reserves vanish.[600]

To those who would turn to aluminum to replace steel the situation is even darker. Aluminum output has grown at about 8% per year in recent years and if this continues, currently economical ore reserves will vanish in about 30 years. And since copper reserves are lower than aluminum, copper alloys of aluminum will no doubt slip from markets sooner.[601]

The attitude that "science will save us" is no longer tenable and never has been true. The use of low grade ores may prolong the lives of certain industries, but claims that we can tax such sources as oceans for minerals are founded on the frightening assumption of the availability of unlimited power. Energy itself is polluting, and the lower the ratio of useful metal to waste matter, the greater the pollution, so turning to inefficient resources promises only to make eventual readjustment more difficult, if not impossible. The idea of using the ocean for minerals is analogous to using antifreeze to make martinis when the gin runs out, and if the era of consumption is not halted by a new set of values, then wars or the life-destroying pollution will bring an end to the era in the lifetimes of today's youth.[602]

The most vulnerable people to the end of the consumption era are the city dwellers, whose primary skills are administrative, sales-oriented or clerical. "Country living" training programs should be made available to everyone so that all of us would have the opportunity to learn to live fundamentally and gratefully.[603]

There is certainly no need to abandon technology. Technological developments can enhance the quality of life for even the self-sufficient farmer. With the aid of scientists, crops could be chosen from the most promising hybrids; methods of clearing land, plowing, tilling, planting, plant production and harvesting could be selected on the basis of a careful balance between imputs and constraints; structures could represent the synthesis of architectural and engineering skill; and the mode of transport for market crops and exports could be chosen so as to minimize input of resources. Use of nonpolluting methods and various sized operations will require a great deal of research and experimentation. Innovations in machinery and equipment are in keeping with scales of operations ranging from a single acre to hundreds of acres and using everything from human peddling to steam boilers for power.[604]

Nutritional research should be centered on human studies in which expected improvements, rather than shortcomings, are tested. Vitamin B_{12} needs a carefully watched long-term study and algae, sprouts, greens and edible wild leaves should also be studied carefully.[605]

The return to ecological farming would make it possible to establish 100 million or more small farms, with up to half a billion residents. Thus the opportunity to offer immigration rights to Asians, Latin Americans, Africans and Europeans would arise. The ties of these peoples to their birthland should foster worldwide understanding. Aggression wanes when persons take simple, whole-foods diets and inward peace has no bounds.[606]

A switch to a simple diet would clearly bring an end to the problem of feeding the world during the next two to three decades. After that it would be the job of individuals to limit the number of children to two. The longest-living most sane-eating groups in the world seem to have been close to natural answers to the "population explosion." It behooves us to follow their example rather than foisting off the most wretched part of our own diet, namely pills.[607]

The Government has served agribusiness and resource exploitation for two hundred years. There is now a growing interest in life, as opposed to leisure, people rather than power, and nature's laws, which do justice to all. Steak and white wine in a suburban fortress, protected by armed police, German shepherds and alarm systems, are goals worthy of beasts. Sterile offices, titles and sicophanting subordinates are dismal substitutes for the love and respect of a family. The presupposition that Americans have found a desirable way of life and are healthy, or that sickness, aging, aggression, greed and self-agrandizement are inevitable, must be replaced with a truth emanating from humility. We face a choice of continuing our way until the planet is destroyed or our children are left sick in a nightmare of barren wastes and oilslicks, or of changing our way of life and eating, so we can know peace, our planet can support us and our children can love and respect us.[608]

appendix
I / the SGA diet

INTRODUCTION

The SGA diet, so named for Sprouts, Greens and Algae, is a whole-foods strict vegetarian (vegan) primarily raw foods diet which is designed to give high yet not excessive amounts of all of the required nutrients with a minimum of those factors which contribute to ill health. Calorie for calorie, humans have never, as far as is known, eaten a diet of comparable quality. Arguments against such a diet are twofold; first, it is said strict vegetarian diets containing no oil or oil-rich foods like nuts contain so much bulk that they may cause injury to the lower digestive tract; and second, it is said people just won't eat such things as greens and sprouts when conventional foods are available. To the first argument, the answer is simply that years of trial have resulted in no digestive problems in anyone taking the SGA diet. Indeed those who had previous digestive problems have seen these brought to an end and it is finally being recognized that bulk (or roughage, or fiber as it is variously known) is a vital nutrient which is debilitatingly low in normal diets. To the second argument, it should be made clear that the SGA diet is for those who choose to eat to live, rather than living to eat.

The basis of the SGA diet is up to a pound and a half of raw greens and the same amount of raw sprouts (especially soy sprouts) per day for women and up to two pounds of both sprouts and greens for men. Rounding out the basics of the SGA diet is a fraction of an ounce of seaweed or other algae and to the basics (greens, sprouts and algae) are added a wide variety of plant foods. The type, amount, acquisition and preparation of the basis of the SGA diet, (greens, sprouts and algae) will be discussed in detail. To date, however, no one taking the SGA diet has relied strictly on the basics.

FOOD ENERGY

Because two pounds of greens and two pounds of sprouts provides as little as 600 calories some additional form of food energy is needed. Some have turned to raw fruits alone or raw fruit and nuts to compliment the SGA basics. On the other hand, baked Irish potatoes or yams (hot or cold) make a fine complement to sprouts and greens. Some individuals have used unsalted, oil-free whole wheat bread or unsalted cooked brown rice and other grains for calories. The opportunity for experimentation is vast. Possibilities include winter squashes, special root plants like burdock (which is delectable raw), cheese-like algae (to be discussed) and countless other plant foods.

GREENS

There is an untold variety of highly nutritious green leaf vegetables. The only weak green leafy vegetables are unfortunately the most common ones, namely lettuce, cabbage and green onions. Other familiar green vegetables, especially parsley and collards, are quite strong, nutritionally. In choosing greens one should include those which one enjoys raw, but there are many wonderful greens with which to experiment. Cultivated greens which are commonly used in raw salads include:

Parsley
Watercress
Chard
Endive
Packchoy (Chinese Cabbage)
Spinach

A number of excellent wild greens are also used in conventional raw salads. These tend to be exceptionally good sources of riboflavin and include:

Comfrey
Cress
Pokeweed (Poke)
Purslane leaves
Swamp cabbage ("Skunk" cabbage)

A number of other greens are familiar to many people, but they are very seldom taken raw. Nevertheless they are very satisfying and vastly richer in vitamin content when eaten raw. There are no finer foods in the world than raw "soul food" greens which include:

Rutabaga greens
Collards
Turnip greens
Mustard greens

To the list of Soul foods can be added okra, which is remarkably satisfying raw. Other common greens which are normally cooked but are succulent when eaten raw include:

Kale
Mustard spinach

Broccoli (including the leaves)
Spinach beet leaves
Venespinach
Taro leaves

Among a large number of wild, edible greens that are needlessly cooked are:

Dandelion
Lambsquarter
Dock
Amaranth

This only scratches the surface of world of green leaves. It is safe to assume that any edible dark green leaf is a worthy addition to any diet. Lettuce and cabbage probably began as fine greens, but declined through efforts to increase yields. It is thought that cabbage began as kale and took its present form only after a long history of cultivation.

There is nothing more wholesome or more beautiful than a garden with rows of broad, massive green leaves. The joy of picking and partaking of your own is the joy of living, but for the time being at least, many of us must depend on retail outlets. Unfortunately, many "natural food" stores offer only lettuce, cabbage, tomatoes, carrots, etc., and shun the strong greens because "people just don't buy them." If those who manage these outlets would eat the greens themselves, however, there is little doubt they would offer them and actively encourage customers to buy them. And this should motivate farmers to grow greens without chemicals.

Until natural food outlets see the (green) light and organically grown greens become more plentiful, many of us will have to depend on supermarket greens.

Fresh collards, chard, turnip greens, parsley, broccoli, etc., are readily available. Even conventionally grown greens provide an array of vitamins and minerals that no other foods can match regardless of how they are grown. This is not to say organically grown greens are not to be preferred over chemically grown ones. In no foods is there a more striking difference in taste between those naturally grown (organically grown greens are usually sweet and succulent) and those artificially grown (which tend to be bitingly hot or somewhat tasteless).

Too often there is scant supply of fresh greens in supermarkets but parsley, which is so prolific that growers seldom bathe it with herbicides, pesticides, etc., seems always to be available. Do not hesitate to eat a big bunch or even two bunches of parsley at a single meal.

A far surer, safer and better way to get parsley is, of course, to grow your own. Once started, the plant is prolific to the extent it quickly replaces what is cut away. All greens tend to quickly replace leaves that are cut away, and it is a good idea to get some greens planted or at least make arrangements to buy someone else's organically grown greens.

There is no harm in mixing as many different greens as one sees fit, and there is no upper limit on the amount of greens one should eat. Indeed the SGA diet calls for eventually eating up to two pounds of raw greens per day. Greens can be cut up in conventional salad fashion, then be eaten alone or mixed with sprouts. Until individuals develop a strong liking for greens themselves, they may want to add things like tomatoes to their greens or to use some sort of "dressing." Conventional salad dressings are not in keeping with the SGA diet but less extreme dressings include lemon, lime or other juices, cut up vegetables or fruits, the pulp from juicing, chopped up baked yams, oilseeds or nuts (in small quantities), herbs, powdered kelp (or some other seaweeds), or anything of a vegetable nature that is salt-free, low in oil and is not an extract. A dressing might include a little raw sesame butter, raisins, maple syrup, or any of a number of spices. The main thing is to find a way to enjoy raw greens and then to eat lots of them.

Greens are frequently eaten with a baked potato or yam: the tuber serves the normal role of bread. Most people find plain baked potatoes are one of the best tasting and most satisfying foods they have ever eaten. Hopefully someone will soon write a noncook book dealing with greens.

The seasonality of greens may make it difficult to always find a plentiful supply. In cold climates, locally grown fresh greens are unavailable during the winter which is the peak production period for greens in mild climates. The people living in cold areas can either buy greens grown in milder climates, use dried greens (which have lost lots of vitamins but still have a full supply of minerals) with their sprouts or simply increase their intake of sprouts. Inhabitants of mild climates may find cultivated greens in short supply during the summer and early fall but wild greens or herbs can take up the slack. Those who live in hot climates normally have a year-round supply of dark green leafy vegetables.

SPROUTS

Sprouts are nothing more than young plants. This does not mean, however, that one must plant seeds to obtain sprouts. All that is necessary is to soak seeds overnight and then pour off the water and let them set in a damp cloth covered jar, or bowl or in a so-called "sprouter" which costs about as much as a single steak dinner and lasts indefinitely. After soaking, the seeds should be washed intermittently (say twice a day) until they are fully sprouted. The washings take only seconds and the sprouts can be eaten anytime after the appearance of shoots from the seeds. There is a great deal to be gained vitamin-wise, though, by letting the shoots gain size for a couple of days: even with this the whole process normally takes only two to five days. However, sprouts will eventually go bad if they are not eaten or refrigerated.

Possibly the richest food in the world nutritionally is soybean sprouts. But beginners beware: Soybeans are very difficult to sprout as they tend to sour. It is far better to begin with seeds that are easy to sprout such as:

Mung Beans (*light and crisp*)

Wheat (*something completely different in taste: excellent*)

Triticale (*a little shy of wheat sprouts, taste-wise*)

Alfalfa (*stringy and ideal for salads*)

Rye (*excellent for variety*)

Lentils (*a taste that's addictive*)

Almost all beans are easy to sprout: the dry beans you find in supermarkets are ready for soaking, but it is far better to get organically grown beans. Organically grown beans, grains and other seeds are readily available at virtually all natural food outlets and many health food stores. A word of warning though. Brown rice, buckwheat groats and "whole" oats will not sprout. You need to get all three with the outer husk. Millet, like soybeans, tends to be difficult to sprout. Corn is an interesting seed to sprout but the author has had experience with it.

When sprouting beans you will find a thin, pliable coating tends to separate from the seed, often during soaking virtually always by the time the sprouts are ready for eating. It is best to wash away this coating for the absence of this cover not only enhances the taste of the sprouts but gives a big boon to the quantity of minerals available.

Unless you are a real purist, you may want to go ahead and use tap water for washing the seeds during sprouting. But the initial soaking should be done in spring water, well water or some other water that has escaped science's answers to disease and tooth decay. For the water in which seeds are soaked is taken up by the seeds and is carried by the sprouts.

It is very important to "sprout your own" but if you plan to begin the SGA diet or simply to make sprouts a major part of your diet, you may want to buy a sizable portion of your sprouts, at least until your own output will meet your needs. And you may be able to buy soy sprouts, which are a chore for beginners. Good places to look for mung and soy sprouts are Chinese food stores. If you live in a smaller community and find no Chinese food stores listed, you might contact any Chinese restaurants in the area: where there's Chinese food there's eggroll and where there's eggroll there's sprouts. If the restaurant has them shipped from afar, you may be able to buy them from the restaurant; if he has a local supplier you may be able to buy direct.

The opportunity for sprouting and selling your sprouts seems to be very good. Alfalfa sprouts, and to some extent mung sprouts, are available in many supermarkets. But prices are needlessly high, the seeds are not organic, the water is halidated and often the sprouts are old, if not turning.

However and whenever you get sprouts you get fantastic food. Taken raw, soybean sprouts, bean sprouts and grain sprouts have an unmatched array of strong amounts of vitamins, minerals and protein. During seasons when greens are in short supply, sprouts can take up the gap and alone serve as the basis for a superb diet.

As part of the SGA diet, sprouts can be included in a salad of greens or eaten from a separate bowl. Most people find raw sprouts delectable so there is little problem in adapting to them. The full strength of the SGA diet can be felt with a daily intake of about half a pound of soybean sprouts, up to a half pound of wheat (or some other grain) sprouts and a half pound or more of mung (or some other bean) sprouts. The main points are to take lots of sprouts, and if possible to include soy sprouts in the diet.

If you have greens on hand, they are best eaten at the same meal with your sprouts. Although there is no nutritional advantage to *physically* mixing the two, the mix does, in the minds of most, improve the taste of greens.

ALGAE

Algae are primitive plants that contain chlorophyll but have no true leaves, stems or roots. The most common algae are the vast quantities of free-floating plankton that inhabit the world's waters, so-called "seaweeds" such as kelp, dulse and kombu and the pond scums and "mosses" of fresh water.

Individuals beginning the SGA diet need not concern themselves with algae until they have spent two or three months getting used to greens and sprouts: the body's stores of the nutrients which motivated the inclusion of algae in the SGA diet can carry individuals accustomed to animal products for many months, if not years. There may not be any need for algae in the SGA diet, but there is no harm in taking some and for now at least, there is real risk in assuming one doesn't need the nutrients in algae.

There are two specific (and at least two auxiliary) reasons for including algae in the SGA diet. First and foremost is the fact that algae contain modest to high amounts of vitamin B_{12} whereas sprouts and greens are thought to contain little or no vitamin B_{12}. Second is the fact that seaweeds, at least, contain incredible amounts of iodine in which plant foods grown in iodine-poor soil tend to be low. Other reasons for adding algae to the diet include the unprecedented array of minerals they contain, and the well known fact that algae are potentially one of the most abundant sources of food in the world.

Some seaweeds are exceptionally rich in vitamin B_{12}. An ounce of kombu, which is the most widely used seaweed in Japan, dry weight should cover a week's needs for B_{12}. A fraction of an ounce of any seaweed once a month will more than cover an individual's iodine needs.

Most Americans and Europeans are all too accustomed to taking vast amounts of salt, and since salt is strictly forbidden in the SGA diet, salty tasting seaweed tends to be a real treat for those beginning the SGA diet. Very popular are powdered kelp and dulse "tea" (which is nothing more than finely chopped dulse) which can be used to season greens and sprouts. Both kelp and dulse are North American seaweeds: kelp usually comes from the California coast and dulse from New Brunswick. There are additional seaweeds harvested in Scotland, if not elsewhere in the British Isles.

It can be argued that seaweed is not a natural food for those living inland. In a sense, this is true but bringing a pound or two of seaweed per person per year inland is not likely to dismantle the world's ecological balance: one trainload of seaweed could take care of the entire population of Chicago for a year (and help to bring an end to thousands of trainloads of cattle going in and cattle corpses coming out of Chicago). On the other hand, seaweed is not the only vitamin B_{12}-rich algae. Blue-green algae from fresh waters served as an important part of the diet of the Aztecs. The Aztecs raked the "pond scum" from at least one large lake, Lake Tezcoco and allowed the harvest to dry in the sun whereupon they had a product not unlike cheese in taste and texture. Lake Chad, in Africa, is still used as a source of algae for food. A flat cake called Dike which is derived from fresh water algae is a delicacy in Fort Tamy and other parts of central Africa. We could benefit greatly from the exploration of algae in our own lakes and ponds.

The main reason for including algae in the SGA diet is to provide a source of vitamin B_{12}: it takes as little as an ounce of seaweed per year to cover iodine needs, and in most areas there is plenty of iodine in greens and seeds alone. And where the soil is low in iodine, adding a little kelp to the soil will effect an increase in iodine in the food. Individuals can avoid the use of algae and still get all of the benefit of the SGA diet by eating a couple of ounces of the roots of tomato plants, leeks, collards, etc. Stringy roots derive vitamin B_{12} from microorganisms in the soil so if roots are used as a source of B_{12}, it is most important the growing be organic. Manure abounds with B_{12} as does healthy soil but chemicals retard the growth of microorganisms.

It is quite possible we will learn that no algae or other concentrated source of vitamin B_{12} is needed tò complement the greens and sprouts in the SGA diet. Long time vegans rarely show any signs of B_{12} deficiency and few if any, long-time vegans are taking large amounts of greens and sprouts.

There is no danger in foregoing a B_{12} source for three months or so, but after that, algae or some other source of B_{12} should be included as a regular part of the diet. Many British vegans use a B_{12} supplement derived from microorganisms, and we simply do not know enough about obtaining B_{12} from the intestinal flora to do anything but take a source of the vitamin for now. Those who, for reasons the author does not condone, choose to ignore B_{12} needs should at least get a blood test every six months or so to make sure serum B_{12} levels stay well above the range where there is danger of pernicious anemia.

appendix
II / fruit and nuts diet

Fruit and nut diets are very popular among vegetarians, and there is much to be said for such regimes. Arguments for relying on fruit and nuts are both philosophical and nutritional. Surprisingly the essence of standard philosophical arguments for fruit and nuts hold for the basics of the SGA (sprouts, greens and algae) diet also. And broadening these arguments leads to the conclusion that the SGA basics actually have some philosophical advantages to fruit and nuts; the SGA basics are certainly superior nutritionally. Those who rely on fruit and nuts would do well to add a little algae to their diet and to replace some, if not all, of their nut intake by sprouts of soybeans, legumes and grain seeds and to include some dark green vegetables in their diets. We shall begin our look at fruit and nuts with the philosophy motivating such a diet.

PHILOSOPHICAL ARGUMENTS

Fruit and nut proponents are quick to point out they live off the offerings of trees, and in so doing they do not destroy the plants that feed them. Trees are indeed a natural part of nature's self but so are weeds (or leaf vegetables as we call them upon cultivation). And when we take the larger leaves of collards, mustard greens, parsley, turnip greens, etc. we do not destroy the plant. The plant quickly replenishes its lost leaves and the smaller leaves left to grow do exactly that. Grains are harvested not in the prime of life but at the end of their one season of life. But the purist may be assured grains could be harvested without cutting the stalk since only the seeds are of interest. The same is true of soybeans, beans and peas.

Plants which are uprooted for food include root vegetables and tubers. But such edibles retain the essence of life for potatoes, onions, parsnips, etc. will all sprout if left to rest or soaked in water.

There are few if any vegetarians who live entirely off of the offerings of trees. To do so means foregoing all vegetables, strawberries, grapes, peanuts and other legumes, various oilseeds, grains, honey, grasses, melons, etc. And living off of trees is dubious ethically. For certainly the purist would want to eat from the foods grown in his own region and that can make living off of trees very difficult.

Few are the readers who live in an area where bananas are grown. They are not grown in Europe, populated oceana or North America. Nor are Brazil nuts, cashews, coconuts, papaya, avocados or pineapples grown in these areas. Few of us live in regions where oranges, grapefruit, lemons and pecans are grown. Even our grapes, peaches, pears and strawberries tend to come from concentrated areas to the south of most of us. The preservation, handling and transport of fruit and nuts is a mammoth, resource depleting, polluting process: a half dozen pieces of fruit a day amounts to almost half a ton of fruit a year. On the other hand local tubers, leaf vegetables, seeds or even fruit are excellent bargains ethically and ecologically.

The ethical arguments against nuts and trees are first that yields are two: when the years growers must wait for trees to bear are taken into account yields per acre are of the order of 300 to 500 pounds per acre edible food. Potatoes, for example, might be expected to yield 20,000 pounds per acre. Even when the lower caloric content of potatoes is taken into account, the yield from potatoes is five to ten times as great as that for nuts. Nuts from trees tend to be a luxury food and as such are difficult to defend, ethically.

In spite of the drawbacks cited, fruit and nuts have some important attributes. They are a concentrated food source, that is, they offer more calories per ounce than most leaf vegetables and sprouts. Fruit and nuts can be eaten raw. And, very importantly, people are familiar with fruits and nuts and enjoy them. These points, especially the fact that fruit and nuts are a concentrated source of calories suggests they might serve as the primary source of calories for an SGA-type diet. Or they might supplement the calories of potatoes and/or other tubers. This raises the question as to just how good fruit and nuts are nutritionally and takes us to the next topic.

NUTRITIONAL CONTENT OF FRUIT AND NUTS

It is possible to choose a fruit and nut diet which is fairly strong in terms of content of most vitamins and minerals. However, fruit and nuts tend to be high in fat and somewhat low in protein and a number of vitamins. They contain no vitamin B_{12} and have fairly low quantities of several minerals. They tend to carry an excess of phosphorus, particularly as phytic acid which threatens to raise the risks of deficiencies of at least two minerals. One of the greatest drawbacks of a fruit and nut diet is that the adequacy of a number of vitamins and at least two key minerals depends on specific choices of fruits and nuts.

For clarity, consider a diet consisting of the following:

Food Item	Amount
Almonds	100 grams
Brazil nuts	50 grams
Walnuts	50 grams
Dried figs	100 grams
Dried apricots	50 grams
Dried currants	50 grams
Bananas	3 medium sized
Oranges	2 medium sized
Apples	2 medium sized

For convenience this will be called the FN diet. The FN diet offers 2230 calories with a high 124 grams of fat and only 49 grams of protein. And with the use of other tree-grown nuts to replace the almonds protein levels would fall to about 40 grams. The 124 grams of fat in the FN diet is below average fat levels of Western diets, but it constitutes more than 50% of calories which is above the Western average. However, the low protein content of the diet should offset the high fat to the extent of preventing obesity and reducing the danger of some other fat-related disorders. There seems to be no way to reduce the fat in the FN diet without cutting protein to questionable levels or utilizing foods other than tree-grown nuts or fruit.

Though the FN mix contains a surplus of thiamin, it would contain less than adequate amounts of thiamin without the inclusion of Brazil nuts and oranges. Niacin levels are above minimum requirements but depend critically on the use of almonds and bananas. The caloric content of the FN diet is associated with a riboflavin need of about 1.3 milligrams per day for normal adults and 1.85 milligrams during pregnancy. The diet actually contains 1.65 milligrams, but the elimination of almonds would cut that to only .73 milligrams of riboflavin which represents overt deficiency. Thus, Brazil nuts, bananas and oranges are not readily replaceable by other fruits and nuts and, almonds are absolutely essential not only for protein but also for B-vitamins, especially riboflavin.

Almonds also serve as a primary source of calcium and iron in the FN diet. Without almonds the mix would contain a marginal 400 milligrams of calcium and less than 15 milligrams of iron which is too low for women during pregnancy and marginal during other periods. The critical nature of specific foods in the FN diet extends to apricots for without apricots the FN diet would contain less than half of an adult's needs for vitamin A. There are alternative sources of vitamin A, however. Melons, peaches and to a lesser extent dried prunes contain fair amounts of the vitamin.

The FN diet is rich in magnesium, manganese, copper and potassium.

On the other hand, nuts are very high in phytic acid which tends to render manganese and copper as well as molybdenum and zinc unavailable to the body. This is especially important in the cases of zinc and molybdenum for the FN diet is very low in both. It is difficult to overcome the lack of zinc and molybdenum in fruit and nut diets because fruits are poor sources of both minerals, and nuts would not be outstanding sources even if they were free of phytic acid. Fruit and nut diets also tend to be quite low in iodine and somewhat low in selenium, chromium and possibly vanadium.

The FN diet contains a very fine surplus of pyridoxine (vitamin B_6), but it shows some weakness in other vitamins. It contains only about 3.5 milligrams of pantothenic acid which puts it on a par with the Fitness diet (see Chapter 6) in offering about 50% of needs. The level of biotin is only a small fraction of needs. Biotin can and is synthesized by a strong colony of intestinal bacteria but just how fruit and nuts affect bacteria in the intestines seems not to have been studied. High fat and high quantities of simple carbohydrates (in refined form at least) do adversely affect the vitamins available from synthesis in the intestines. The FN diet is anything but high in folacin with a total folacin content of only 177 micrograms. The Food and Nutrition Board recommends 400 micrograms. Distinctly low in the FN diet is vitamin K: needs are for over 0.5 milligrams of vitamin K, but the FN diet contains less than 0.2 milligrams. The FN diet contains a very rich 20 grams of vitamin R (roughage) and 170 milligrams of vitamin C and it is high in vitamin P. It should be noted though that nuts, dried fruits and even many fresh fruits are poor sources of vitamin C and P: without citrus fruit the FN diet would be very low in both vitamins. The FN diet would tend to be a poor source of vitamin B_{17} unless fruit seeds were included in the diet. Unfortunately there seems to be no reliable source of the vitamin E content of nuts. It does appear, however, that the FN diet contains less than 15 milligrams of vitamin E which in view of very high quantities of polyunsaturated fatty acids in general, and linoleic acid in particular, is extremely low. Vitamin B_{15} levels may also be low and there is no vitamin B_{12} in the FN diet.

The most likely deficiencies from the FN diet are vitamin B_{12}, pantothenic acid, biotin, vitamin K, molybdenum, vitamin U, zinc, selenium and iodine. Shortages of vitamin E, folacin, chromium and manganese could also occur. And less delicately chosen fruit and nut diets could be low in calcium, iron, riboflavin, niacin, thiamin, vitamin C, vitamin P, vitamin B_{17} and even protein.

Lack of vitamin B_{12}, molybdenum, iron, folacin and vitamin C are all associated with some form of anemia. Low levels of zinc, iodine, selenium, protein, riboflavin and some other nutrients in which fruit and nut diets tend to be low tend to retard growth and sexual maturity. Deficiencies in pantothenic acid, biotin, vitamin E, niacin and thiamin tend to promote emotional disturbances including apathy, irritability, somnolence, insomnia, depression and general dissatisfaction. Thus a pure fruit and nut diet might be expected to be somewhat ill-suited for children, young women and others wanting to lead active, involved lives.

Supplementing fruit and nuts with greens and sprouts can eliminate every potential deficiency except vitamin B_{12} and iodine while a little seaweed can cover B_{12} and iodine needs. Thus fruit and nuts with a chunk of SGA can provide a complete diet, and a good one. It could improve further, though, by decreasing nut intake and replacing some fruit with vegetables. A fruit and nut diet is markedly improved, in theory at least, by the inclusion of peanuts. But raw peanut protein is thought not to be utilizable so that peanuts should be roasted. This of course defeats the purpose of a raw foods diet, and if one accepts a limited amount of cooked food he might want to consider baked potatoes with his or her fruit, nuts, greens, sprouts and seaweed. The more one moves towards SGA-type diets the stronger the diet becomes.

Fortunately those who adhere to fruit and nuts alone are few. And since seeds, leaf vegetables and algae are at least equally defensible ethically there seems to be little reason to reject strong help from the SGA basics.

appendix
III / cancer mathematics

A PROOF THAT OBESITY BOOSTS CANCER INCIDENCE ALMOST THREEFOLD

Let $p(A,B.../a,b...)$ represent the conditional probability of events A, B,... given the occurrence of events a, b,...

A = an age reached by a policyholder,

W = the weight class of a policyholder and,

A_0 = the age at issuance of policy.

Exhibit 11 gives $p(A/W=normal, A_0=47)$, $p(A/W=25\%$ above normal, $A_0=47)$ and $p(A/W=20\%$ under normal, $A_0=47)$ for $A \geqslant 47$. Exhibit 12 gives $p(A/W, A_0=55)$ for the same three weight classes and $A \geqslant 55$. The figures are based on the assumption the overall mortality rate rises 8.2% per year or about 120% every ten years and uses the life expectancies given in Exhibit 10.

Letting C represent the event of dying of cancer it is clear Exhibit 8 is a compilation of

$$p(C/W,A_0) \qquad [1]$$

A more meaningful measure of the relationship between weight class and vulnerability to cancer would be

$$p(C/W, A_0, A).$$

If W_1 and W_2 are two different weight classes then presumably

$$\frac{p(C/W_1,A_0,A)}{p(C/W_2,A_0,A)} \qquad [3]$$

is independent of A (i.e. if at one age a very overweight man is twice as likely to die of cancer as a lighter man, the same will be true at any later age they both reach.) Define [3] as $r(W_1,W_2,A_0)$.

From elementary probability theory

$$p(C/W,A_0) = \sum_A p(C/W,A_0,A) \, p(A/W,A_0) \qquad [4]$$

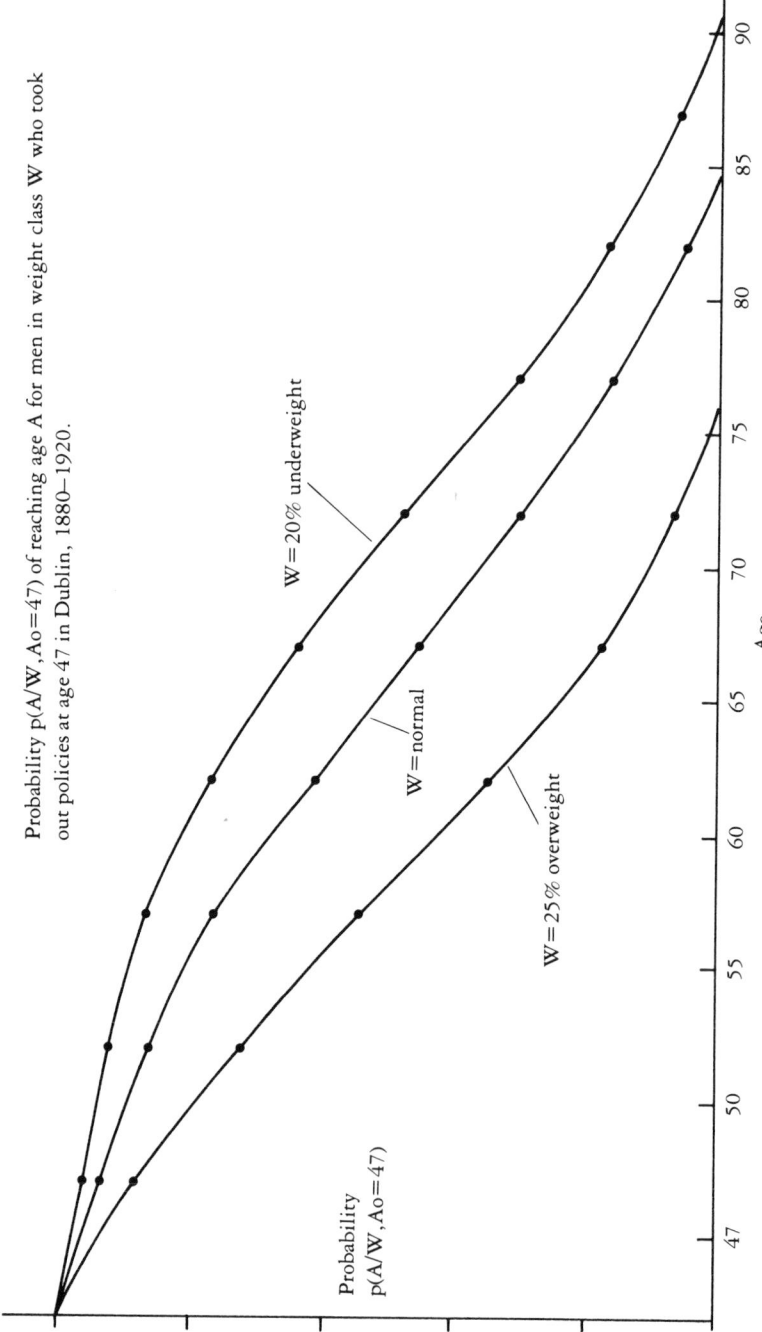

Exhibit 11

Probability p(A/W,Ao=47) of reaching age A for men in weight class W who took out policies at age 47 in Dublin, 1880–1920.

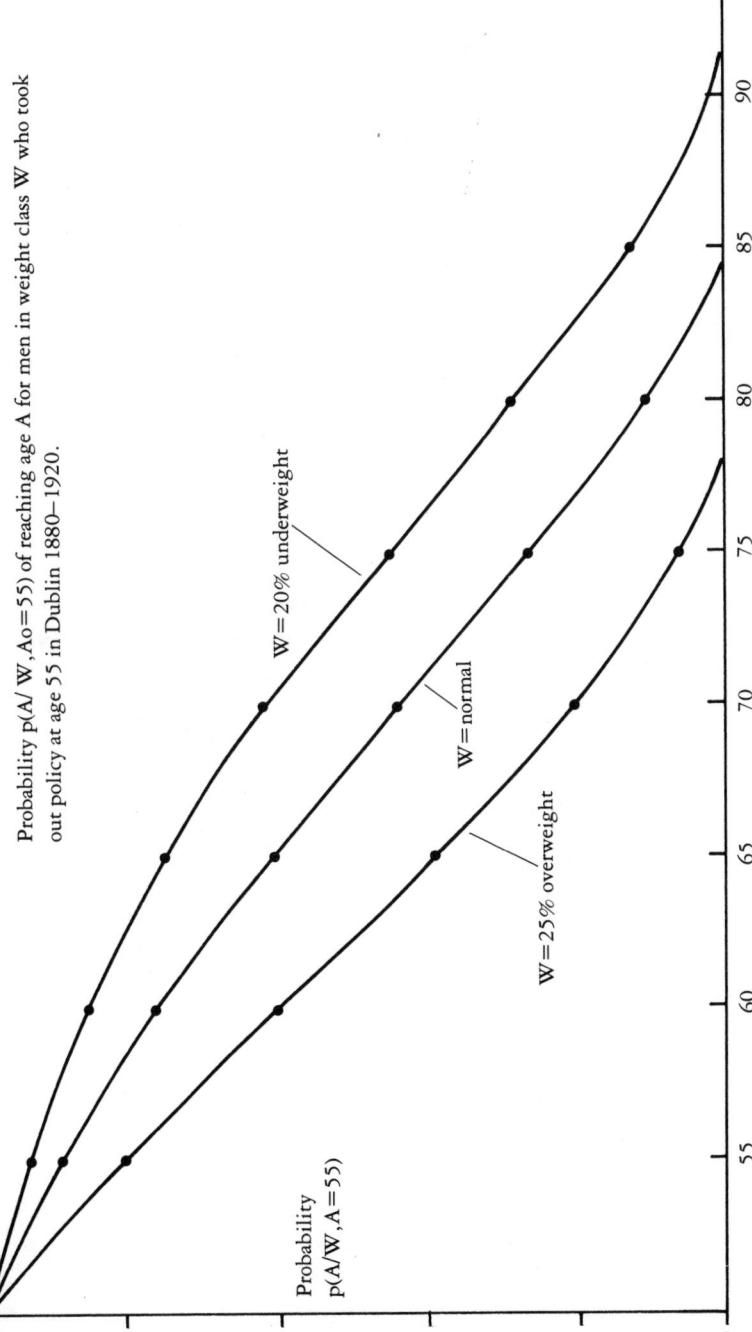

Exhibit 12

Probability p(A/W,Ao=55) of reaching age A for men in weight class W who took out policy at age 55 in Dublin 1880–1920.

W = 20% underweight

W = normal

W = 25% overweight

Probability
p(A/W, A=55)

so putting

$$t(W_1, W_2, A_0) = \frac{p(C/W_1, A_0)}{p(C/W_2, A_0)} \qquad [5]$$

and

$$r(W_1, W_2, A_0) = t(W_1, W_2, A_0) \frac{\sum_A p(C/W_1, A_0, A)\, p(A/W_1, A_0)}{\sum_A p(C/W_2, A_0, A)\, p(A/W_2, A_0)} \qquad [6]$$

Now presumably

$$\frac{p(C/W, A_0, A)}{p(C/W, A_0, A_0)} \qquad [7]$$

is dependent of W, that is the way in which the probability of dying of cancer rises after a (say) $A_0 = 45$ is uniform for all weight groups. Then defining $[7]$ as $v(C/A_0, A)$ we get $[6]$ can be written

$$r(W_1, W_2, A_0) = t(W_1, W_2, A_0) \frac{\sum_A v(C/A_0, A)\, p(A/W_2, A_0)}{\sum_A v(C/A_0, A)\, p(A/W_1, A_0)} \qquad [8]$$

The values of $v(C/A_0 = 47, A)$ for $A \geqslant 47$ and $v(C/A_0 = 55, A)$ for $A \geqslant 55$ are plotted against A in Exhibits 13 and 14 respectively. Thus $p(W = normal, W_2, A_0)$ for $W_2 = 25\%$ overweight, $W_2 = 20\%$ underweight, $A_0 = 47$, $A_0 = 55$ can be computed by $[8]$ using Exhibit C8 for t (normal, W_2, A_0) and exhibits 11 and 12 for $p(A/W_2, A_0)$ and $p(A/$ normal, A_0). Then

$$r(\text{normal}, 25\% \text{ overweight}, A_0 = 47) = 2.85 \qquad [9]$$
$$r(\text{normal}, 25\% \text{ overweight}, A_0 = 55) = 2.42 \qquad [10]$$

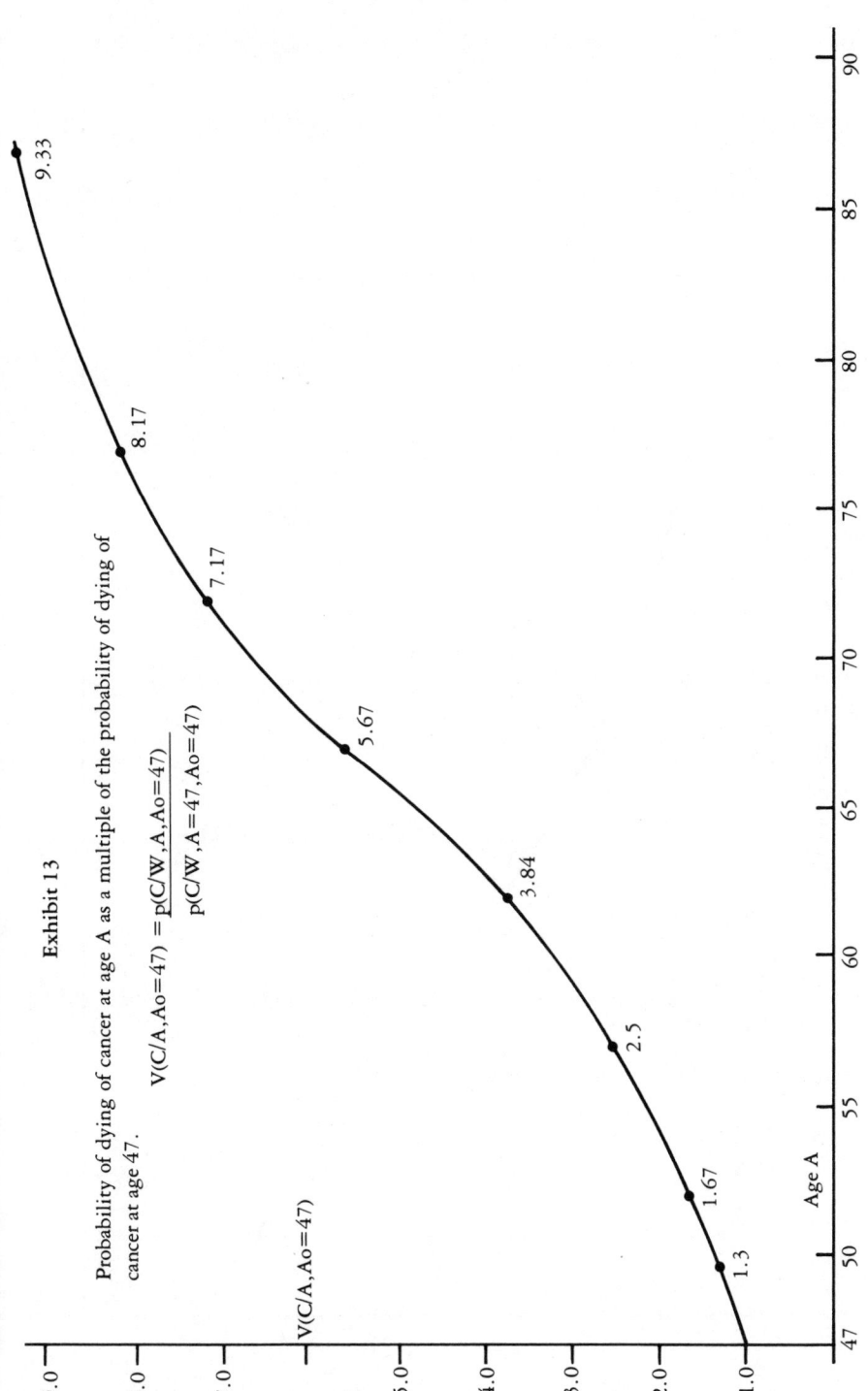

Exhibit 13

Probability of dying of cancer at age A as a multiple of the probability of dying of cancer at age 47.

$$V(C/A, Ao=47) = \frac{p(C/W, A, Ao=47)}{p(C/W, A=47, Ao=47)}$$

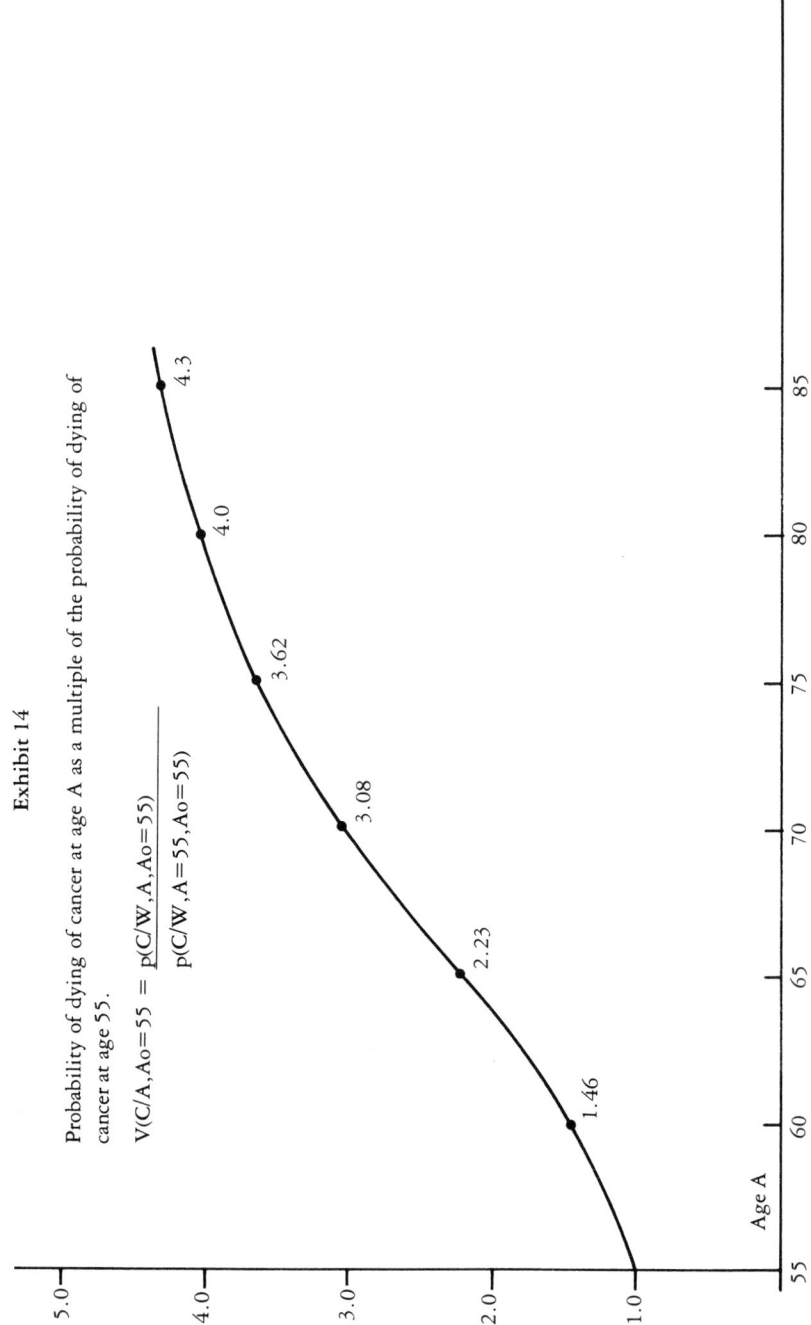

Exhibit 14

Probability of dying of cancer at age A as a multiple of the probability of dying of cancer at age 55.

$$V(C/A, Ao=55) = \frac{p(C/W, A, Ao=55)}{p(C/W, A=55, Ao=55)}$$

Age A

and when $W = 20\%$ underweight, $W = 25\%$ overweight we get

$$r(20\% \text{ underweight, } 25\% \text{ overweight, } 47 \text{ years}) = 3.9 \qquad [11]$$
$$r(20\% \text{ underweight, } 25\% \text{ overweight, } 55 \text{ years}) = 3.4 \qquad [12]$$

Thus assuming the average Union Central policyholder bought his policy before age 55, it appears the age adjusted cancer mortality rate for very obese men is two to three times as great as the rate for men of average weight. The rate for the very obese appears to be three to four times the rate for the very slim.

For a check on these results let d_A represent the act of dying at age A, W_F represent the property of being 25% above normal and W_N represent being of normal weight. Since the cancer mortality rate climbs faster than the overall mortality rate until age sixty-five we have for $A_0 \leqslant A \leqslant 65$.

$$\frac{p(C/W_F,d_A)}{p(C/W_N,d_A)} \geqslant \frac{p(C/W_F,A_0)}{p(C/W_N,A_0)} = 1.29 \qquad [13]$$

the last equality coming from Exhibit 8. Then

$$r(W_F,W_N,A_0) = \frac{p(C/W_F,A_0,A)}{p(C/W_N,A_0,A)} = \frac{p(C/W_F,d_A)p(d_A/W_F,A)}{p(C/W_N,d_A)p(d_A/W_N,A)} \geqslant$$

$$\frac{1.29 \, p(d_A/W_F,A)}{p(d_A/W_N,A)} \qquad [14]$$

but Verdy (44) says

$$\frac{p(d_A/W_F,A)}{p(d_A/W_N,A)} = 1.75 \text{ for all } A, \qquad [15]$$

so that 14 can be evaluated by

$$r(W_N,W_F,A_0) = (1.29) \ (1.75) = 2.25 \qquad [16]$$

which substantiates [9] and [10]. $\qquad [17]$

appendix
IV / vitamins and minerals

Exhibit I gives a summary of the estimated requirements for 19 vitamins. It also gives estimates of normal levels of intake in the U.S., and it lists some recommended sources of each vitamin. It should be noted that the U.S. diet appears to be quite low in vitamin R (roughage), vitamin U, nitrilosides, vitamin K, pyridoxine, biotin, pantothenic acid, vitamin E and folacin. Possible consequences of these shortages include a disturbed emotional state, cancer, intestinal disorders, ulcers, hemorrhaging, anemia, cardiovascular diseases and reproduction maladies. The recommended sources are, in all cases, outstanding sources of the vitamin for which they are recommended. However, they are not, in all cases, the very richest sources of the vitamin in question. Raw liver was left out of several listings because of the excesses (e.g. vitamin A, purines, cholesterol, protein) it would introduce into the diet. Pork and eggs were dismissed from at least two listings because of gross excesses of fat and cholesterol. Note that green leafy vegetables are a recommended source of every vitamin.

Exhibit II gives estimates of requirements for 15 essential minerals and of normal intakes of these minerals. It also lists some good sources of usable supplies of each. It is interesting that plant foods are excellent sources of calcium and phosphorus, potassium, magnesium, manganese, chromium, molybdenum and copper, iron, zinc, fluorine and selenium. Selected animal products are high in copper and zinc, but all animal products are extremely low in magnesium and manganese and tend to be low in chromium and molybdenum as well. Animal products tend to have poor molybdenum-copper ratios, and among animal products only milk derivatives have favorable calcium-phosphorus ratios or a good supply of calcium. It is often said a "mixed" diet is best. This is true in the sense that leaf vegetables could be selected for their high content of calcium, iron, magnesium, manganese, molybdenum and potassium, and complemented by sprouts of soybeans, beans and grains which offer high levels of available potassium, magnesium, zinc, iron, copper, molybdenum, manganese, chromium, fluorine and selenium. With the addition of a little seaweed to the mix of greens and sprouts, one gets 1) the SGA "mix" and 2) a high level of every mineral believed to be necessary for humans. There is nothing to be gained by adding anything of animal origin.

Exhibit I

Estimated Needs for Vitamins

VITAMIN	BASIC REQUIREMENT PER DAY				NORMAL INTAKE IN U.S.	RECOMMENDED SOURCES
	INFANT	CHILD	NORMAL ADULT	PREGNANT OR LACTATING WOMEN		
C	20–25 mg	up to 90 mg	90 mg	115 mg/day	50–70 mg/day	Green leafy vegetables
A	2000 IU/day	up to 5000 IU	3000–4000 IU	over 6000 IU/day	over 4000 IU per day for those taking good vegetable sources	Green leafy vegetables; liver may be excessive.
Folacin (folic acid)	40 micrograms	up to 100 micrograms free folacin	100 micrograms free folacin	200 micrograms free folacin	under 40 µg	Sprouted soybeans, beans and grains, leaf vegetables.
Cobalamin	0.2 micrograms	up to 0.3 micrograms	0.3 micrograms	0.5 micrograms	over 3 micrograms	Seaweed, milk, fatty fish, roots of vegetables, fresh water algae, comfrey and sprouts
D	4–8 IU from human milk	up to 400 IU	over 100 IU	over 100 IU	over 400 IU for those taking vit. D supplemental products	Direct exposure to lots of sunshine, fatty fish, sundried powdered mushrooms.
E (d-alpha-tocopherol)	0.9 mg/gPUFA normally; 0.3 mg/gPUFA if linolic acid intake low.	0.9 mg/gPUFA normally; 0.3 mg/gPUFA if linolic acid intake low.	0.9 mg/gPUFA normally; 0.3/gPUFA if linolic acid intake low.	0.9 mg/gPUFA normally 0.3/gPUFA if linolic acid intake low.	0.2 mg/gPUFA but fairly low in linolic acid	Green leafy vegetables, sprouted wheat, sprouted soybeans, oilseeds and nuts.
Riboflavin (vitamin B$_2$)	0.5 mg/1000 cal.	0.7 mg/1000 cal.	0.6 mg/1000 cal.	0.8 mg/1000 cal.	over 0.6 mg per 1000 cal. for those taking more than two or more glasses of milk	Green leaf vegetables, sprouts, milk, fatty fish and raw eggs.

Thiamin (vitamin B$_1$)	0.3 mg/1000 cal.	0.4 mg/1000 cal.	0.5 mg/1000 cal.	probably under 0.4 mg/1000 cal.	Sprouts, all vegetables, especially green ones.
Niacin	3–5 mg/1000 cal.	6 mg/1000 cal.	6 mg/1000 cal.	probably over 7 mg/1000 cal.	Fish, sprouts, green vegetables, most whole foods.
Pantothenic acid	3 mg/1000 cal.	3 mg/1000 cal.	4 mg/1000 cal.	probably under 2 mg/1000 cal.	Vegetables and sprouts.
Biotin	about 11 µg/1000 cal.	up to 50 µg/1000 cal.	up to 50 µg/1000 cal.	Very low for those taking high levels of refined foods.	Grain sprouts, milk, fatty fish, chicken and vegetables.
Pyridoxine (vitamin B$_6$)	15 µg/g protein on low protein intake, 30 µg/g protein otherwise.	15 µg/g protein on low protein intake, 30 µg/g protein otherwise.	15 µg/g protein on low protein intake, 30 µg/g protein otherwise.	about 15 µg/1000 cal. with high protein intake.	All plant foods.
K	probably under .5 mg/day	.5–2.0 mg per day	.5–2.0 mg per day	very low	Green leaf vegetables.
P				Very low if lacking fresh fruits and vegetables	Plant foods, especially buckwheat and vitamin C-rich fruits and vegetables.
Pangamic Acid (Vitamin B$_{15}$)	not estb.	not estb.	not estb.	May be low	Plant foods.
Nitrilosides (Vitamin B$_{17}$)	not estb.	not estb.	not estb.	Probably very low	Seeds from fruit, sprouts, green leaf vegetables.
U	not estb.	not estb.	not estb.	Low	Green leafy vegetables, cauliflower, and cabbage.
R (fiber)	10 g/day	10 g/day	10 g/day	Under 6 g/day and inadequate	Whole plant foods
Orotic Acid (Vitamin B$_{13}$)	not estb.	not estb.	not estb.	May be low	Vegetables, especially beets and other root vegetables, milk.

Exhibit II

Dietary Materials

	RECOMMENDED DAILY INTAKE			ESTIMATED DAILY INTAKE IN	
MINERAL	INFANT	CHILD	ADULT	U.S.	SOURCES
Calcium	300 mg	300 mg/ 1000 cal. and more than 400 mg total	400–500 mg per day	over 600	Green leafy vegetables, broccoli, okra, milk, sesame, seeds, blackstrap molasses, peel of citrus fruit, cheese.
Phosphorus	100 mg	400 mg	Ca:P ratio 1:1.5	Ca:P approx. 1:3	Green leafy vegetables, offer most favorable Ca:P ratio: meat, eggs, fish, and fowl tend to put an excess of phosphorus in diet, lower Ca:P.
Sodium and Chlorine as Salt	none	none	none	10–20 g salt/day	All whole foods have adequate supply of sodium and chlorine; animal products tend to provide an excess.
Potassium	300 mg K and K:Na ratio over 1.0	Total K 600 mg, and K:Na ratio over 1.0	Total K over 1000 mg and K:Na over 1.0	K:Na ratio under 0.2	Soybeans, beans, whole grains, vegetables and fruits all high in K with favorable K:Na.
Magnesium	about 10 mg/kg body weight	up to 10 mg/kg body weight	over 5 mg/kg body weight	about 3 mg/ kg	Whole grains, beans, peas, soybeans, nuts, and green leafy vegetables.
Zinc	3 mg.	6–9 mg.	6 mg. free Zn.	6–12 mg. Zn.	Sprouted beans, organ meats, shellfish, mushrooms, parsley, kale
Copper	.4 mg.	1-2 mg.	2 mg.	low for many	Sprouted beans, organ meats, shellfish, mushrooms, parsley, kale

Exhibit II (continued)

Iron	under 1 mg	girls 20 mg	25 mg for normal women 30 mg during pregnancy and lactation	pregnant women under 20 mg., girls under 15 mg	Green leafy vegetables, soybeans, whole grains, organ meats, blackstrap molasses
Molybdenum	Amount in human milk	600 micrograms or more	600 micrograms and and Cu:Mo less than 3:1	350 micrograms and Cu:Mo often over 5:1	Whole grains, sprouted beans, plant foods
Manganese	Amount in human milk	2–5 mg.	4 mg.	may often be under 1 mg.	Whole grains, beans and nuts; animal products and refined items low.
Iodine	50 micrograms	200 micrograms	300 micrograms	may be low unless taking iodized salt.	Seaweed plant foods grown in iodine-rich soil and seafoods.
Chromium	Amount in human milk	unknown	unknown	very low	Whole grains, beans, other unprocessed plant foods.
Fluorine	Amount in human milk	1 mg or more	1 mg or more	2 mg or more where water treated	Seaweed, soybeans, buckwheat, foods from F rich soil
Selenium	15 micrograms	up to 90 micrograms	90 micrograms	may be under 20 micrograms.	Whole grains, oilseeds.

paragraph references

References: Chapter 1
1. Brooke, B.N. "Understanding Cancer," pp. 6–13, Holt, Rinehart and Winston, 1973.
    Sutton, P.M. "The Nature of Cancer," pp. 19–26, Crowell, 1965.
2. Nowinski, W.W. "Fundamental Aspects of Normal and Malignant Growth," pp. 140, 159, 897, 898, Elsevier, 1960.
    McGrady, P. "The Savage Cell," pp. 1–6, Basic Books, 1964.
3. Hegsted, D.M. in "Nutrition," Vol. I, ed. by Beaton, G.H. and McHenry, E.W., pp. 125–6, Academic Press, 1964.
4. Stump, D.J. Colliers Encyclopedia, 5:342, 1969.
5. Natenberg, M. "The Cancer Blackout," Regent House, 1959.
    Haught, S.J. "Has Dr. Max Gerson a True Cancer Cure?", p. 92, London Press, 1962.
6. Price, W.A. "Nutrition and Physical Degeneration," Am. Acad. of Nutr., 1950.
    Armstrong, Trevor. Soil and Health J. (New Zealand)Oct-Nov., 1965.
    Benet, Sula. Personal Communication. March 8, 1974.
    Schweitzer, A. "How White Man's Diet Affects Natives of Africa," 1954.
8. Preston, S.H., et al. "Causes of Death," Seminar Press, 1972.
    MacDonald, Eleanor J. The Cancer Bulletin (U.Tex.at Houston), 25(2):33, 1973.
9. Cutler, S.J. and Haenszel, W.M. "The Magnitude of the Cancer Problem," Pub.Health Rep., 69:334, 1954; phone conversation with authors during February, 1974.
10. Cutler, S.J. "Report on the 3rd Nat.Cancer Survey," Am.Cancer Society report from 7th Conference Proc., pp. 639–652, 1973.
11. Herber, Lewis. "Our Synthetic Environment," p. 144, Jonathan Cape, 1963.
13. Cutler, S.J. Op.Cit.
14. Tannenbaum, Albert. Ann.NY Acad.Science, 49:10, 1947.
15. Greenstein, J.P. "Biochemistry of Cancer," p. 253, Academic Press, 1954.
    Anderson, D.E., et al. J.Natl.Cancer Inst., 45:697, 1970.

16. Ross, R.H. and Bras, G. J.Nat.Cancer Inst., 47:1095, 1971.
17. Tannenbaum, A., and Silverstone, H. Advances in Cancer Research, 1:452, 1953.

Greenstein, J.P. Op.Cit., p. 257.

18. Hoffman, F.L. "Cancer and Diet," p. 767, Williams and Wilkins, 1937.

Tannenbaum, A. in "The Physiopathology of Cancer," F.Homburge (ed) p. 517, Hoeber, 1959.

deWaard, F. et al. Cancer, 22:988, 1968.

Sneddon, A., et al. Lancet, 2:892, 1968.

Tannenbaum, A. Ann.N.Y.Acad. Sci., 49:15, 1947.

20. Preston, S.H., et al. "Causes of Death," Seminar Press, 1972.

U.S.Dept.Comm., Bureau of the Census, Stat.Abs. of U.S., pp. 53–58, 1970.

Ross, M.H. Am.Journ.Clinical Nutrition, 25:834, 1973.

Verdy, Maurice. Can.J.Public Health, 58:494, 1967.

21. Benet, Sula. New York Times, Dec. 26, 1971.
22. Joliffe, Norman. "Reduce and Stay Reduced," pp. 22–23, Simon & Schuster, 1957.
23. Leveille, G.A., et al. J.Nutr., 93:541, 1967.

Cohn, C., et al. Melab., 6:381, 1957.

Stevenson, J.A.F., et al. Proc.Soc.Exptl.Bio.Med., 116:178, 1964.

Leveille, G.A. and Hanson, R.W. Can.J.of Physiol. and Pharmacology, 43:857, 1965.

Mukaida, C.S. and Lickton, I.J. J.Nutr., 101(6):767, 1971.

Leveille, G.A. J. Nutr., 91(2 pt 1):267, 1967.

24. Schemmel, R., et al. J. Nutr., 102:1187, 1972.

Marshall, Mary, et al. Proc.Soc.Exptl.Bio.Med., 132(1):227, 1969.

28. Vukovic, D. Kinderaerztl.Prax., 40(4):185, 1972.

Passmore, R. Proc.Soc.Nutr., 30:122, 1971.

Balestreri, R. and Bertolini, S. Arch.Maragl.Patol.Clin., 27(2): 45, 1972.

Dudenko, N.V. Op.Okhr.Materin.Det., 14(9):83, 1969.

Gelvin, E.P. and McGavack, T.H. "Obesity, Its Cause, Classification and Care," p. 10, Hoeber-Harper, 1957.

29. Robertson, W. van B. and Kahler, H. J.Natl. Cancer Inst., 2: 595, 1942.

Greenstein, J.P. Op.Cit., pp. 350–353, 516–541, 544.

Rosenfeld, I. and Tobias, C.A. J.Biol.Chem., 191:339, 1951.

30. Abels, J.C. et al. Ann.Internal Med., 16:221, 1942.

Buckner, Nancy and Swaffield, M. Cancer Res., 33(12):3189, 1973.

Greenstein, J.P. Op.Cit., p. 509.

31. Schmeck, H.M. New York Times, June 30, 1961.
    Strong, L.C. "Biological Aspects of Aging," pp. 107–133, 197, Pergom Press, 1968.
    Sloan Kittering Institute for Cancer Research Progress Report XI, p. 14, New York, 1958.

32. D'Ambrosio, J. Branksom Acupuncture Clinic, Kenilworth, England, personal correspondences, 1972–74.
    Bieler, H.G. "Food is Your Best Medicine," p. 172, Vintage Books, 1st Edition, 1972.
    Haught, S.J. Op.Cit., p. 67.

34. DeCarli, L.M. and Lieber, C.S. J. Nutr., 91(3 pt. 1):331, 1967.
    Jones, D.P. and Green, E. Am.J.Clin.Nutr., 18(5):350, 1966.
    Ruben, Emanual. Public Radio Station KUT, "All Things Considered," Austin, Texas, February 3, 1974.
    U.S. Public Health Service. "Smoking and Health," Pub.No. 1103, 1964.
    Staszewski, J. Brit.J.Cancer, 14:419, 1960; 23:247, 1969.
    Chabon, A.B., et al. Cancer, 33:1577, 1974.

35. Chang, M.L.W., et al. J.Nutr., 101(3):323, 1971.
    Durand, A.M.A., et al. Arch.Pathol., 85:318, 1968.
    Kuo, P.T., et al. Am.J.Clin.Nutr., 26:116, 1967.

36. Chalvardjian, A. and Stephens, S. J.Nutr., 100(4):397, 1970.
    Khan, I.H. and Yudkin, J. Proc.Nutr.Soc., 30:74A, 1971.

37. Lavik, P.S. and Baumann, C.A. Cancer Res., 3(11):749, 1943.
    Silverstone, H., et al. Cancer Res., 12(10):750, 1952.
    Ward, J.M., et al. J.Natl.Cancer Inst., 51:713, 1973.

38. Antar, M.A., et al. American Journal of Clinical Nutrition, 14:169, 1964.
    Price, W.A. Op.Cit.
    Armstrong, Trevor. Op.Cit.
    Benet, S. New York Times, December 26, 1971.

39. Hunter, B.T. "Food Additives," Keats, 1972.
    Naismith, D.J., et al. J.Nutr., 97(3):375, 1969.
    Schmauz, R. and Cole, P.J. Natl.Cancer Inst., 52:1431, 1974.
    Ibid. Lancet, 1:1335, 1971.

40. Rudas, B., et al. Nutr. Metab., 15(6):315, 1973.
    Newberne, P.M. and Salmon, W.D. J.Nutr., 79(2):179, 1963.
    Wostmann, B.S. J.Nutr., 103(7):982, 1973.
    Okada, M. and Ochi, A. J.Biochem. (Japan), 70:581, 1971.
    Bergman, F., et al. Acta Pathol.Microbiol.Scand.Pathol.Sect.A., 78:179, 1970.

41. Marshall, M.W. and Hildebrand, H.E. J.Nutr., 79:227, 1963.
De, H.N., et al. Pakistan J. Med.Res., 6:146, 1967.
Chang, M.L.W., et al. J.Nutr., 96(3):368, 1968.
Haught, S.J. Op.Cit., p. 89.
Natenberg, M. Op.Cit., p. 88.
42. Malmros, H., et al. Act.Med.Scand., 192:201, 1972.
Katsumata, K. Nagoya J.Med.Sci., 32:407, 1970.
Naismith, D.J., et al. Proc.Soc.Nutr., 31:94A, 1972.
43. Steiner, P.E. Cancer Res., 2:425, 1942; 3:385, 1943; 7:273, 1947.
Hieger, I. Brit.J.Nutr., 3:123, 1949.
Moll, R. Zool.Anz., 178:18, 1967.
44. Price, W.A. Op.Cit.
Armstrong, Trevor. Op.Cit.
Benet, Sula, Personal Communication, March 8, 1974.
Standard and Poor's Industry Reports, Vol.141(37):1, 1973.
Hirayama, T. "Smoking in Relation to the Death Rates of 265,118 Men and Women in Japan," Nat.Cancer Center, Res.Inst., Tokyo, September, 1967, p. 14.
Ishii, K., et. al. Jap.J.Clin.Med., 26:1839, 1968.
Haenszel, B., et al. J.Natl.Cancer Inst., 51(6):1765, 1973.
Drasar, B.S. and Irving, D. Brit. J. Cancer, 27(2):167, 1973.
Newsweek, p. 80, Feb. 18, 1974.
Benet, S. "Abkhasians," p. 25, Holt, Rinehart and Winston, 1974.
46. Greenstein, J.P. Op.Cit., p. 241.
Kaunitz, H., et al. Z. Ernaehrungswiss, 10:61, 1970.
47. Silverstone, H. and Tannenbaum, A. Cancer Res., 11:200, 1951; 10:448, 1950.
Dunning, W.F., et al. Cancer Res., 9:354, 1949.
Haught, S.J. Op.Cit., pp. 86, 89.
Newsweek, p. 80, Feb. 18, 1974.
Editorial. Cancer News, 25(1):13, 1971.
Stein, J.J. Ibid, 28(1):4, 1974.
New York Post. June 24, 1974.
48. U.S. Publ.Health Ser., NCI. "Survey of Compounds Which Have Been Tested for Carcinogenic Activity," Bethesda, Md., 1951.
Watt, B.K. and Merrill, A.L. "Composition of Foods," USDA Handbook No. 8, 1963.
49. Silverstone, H. and Tannenbaum, A. Cancer Res., 10:448, 1950.
Bishop, J.E. Wall Street Journal, Oct. 23, 1973.
Cook, J.W. and Haslewood, D. J.Chem.Soc., 248, 1948.

50. Greenstein, J.P. Op.Cit., p. 49.
    Frieser, L.F. "Chemistry of Natural Products Related to Phenanthrene," Reinhold, 1936.
    Young, C.W. "The Americana 1972 Annual," p. 443, 1973.
    Wynder, E.L., et. al. Cancer, 20:1520, 1967.
51. Kaunitz, H. et al. Z. Ernaehrungswiss, 10:61, 1970.
    Silverstone, H. and Tannenbaum, A. Cancer Res., 10:448, 1950.
    U.S. Publ.Health Ser., NCI, "Survey of Compounds Which Have Been Tested for Carcinogenic Activity," Bethesda, Md., 1951.
    Boutwell, R.K., et al. Cancer Res., 9:741, 1949.
    Karvonen, M.J. Proc.Nutr.Soc., 31:355, 1972.
    Opie, E.L. "Approaches to Tumor Chemotherapy," Am.Asso. Adv.Sci., p. 125, 1947.
52. Steiner, P.E. Cancer Res., 2:425, 1942; 3:385, 1943; 7:273, 1947.
    Hieger, I. Brit.J.Nutr., 3:123, 1949.
    Siperstein, M.D., et al. Cancer Res., 26:7, 1966.
    Abels, J.C., et al. Ann.Internal Med., 16:221, 1942.
53. Bricker, L.A., Cancer Res., 34:449, 1974.
    Bricker, L.A., et al. J.Clin. Invest., 51:206, 1972.
    Chen, H.W., et al. Cancer Res., 33:2774, 1973.
    Mason, H.L. and Kepler, E.J. J.Biol.Chem., 161:235, 1945.
    Abels, J.C., et al. Ann.Internal Med., 16:221, 1942.
54. Huggins, C. Physiol.Rev., 25:281, 1945.
55. Denbesten, L., et al. Gastroenterology, 66:1036, 1974.
    Mijake, H. and Johnston, C.G. Digestion, 1:219, 1968.
    Kameda, H. Gastroenterology, 46:109, 1964.
    Encly. Brit., 4:770, 1969.
56. Newsweek, p. 80, Feb. 18, 1974.
    Haenszel, B., et al. J.Natl.Cancer Inst., 51(6):1765, 1973.
    Irving, D. and Draser, B.S. Brit.J.Cancer, 28(5):462, 1973.
    Drasar, B.S. and Irving, D. Brit.J.Cancer, 27(2):167, 1973.
57. Ibid.
    Wynder, E.L., et al. Cancer, 13:559, 1960; 20:113, 1967.
    Lea, A.J. Lancet, 2:332, 1966.
    Carroll, K.K., et al. Can.Med.Assoc.J., 98:590, 1968.
58. Hirayama, T. Op.Cit.
    Ishii, K., et al. Jap.J.Clin.Med., 26:1839, 1968.
    Wynder, E.L., et al. J.Natl.Cancer Inst., 50:645, 1973.
59. Greenstein, J.P. Op.Cit., pp. 27–29, 1954.
60. Loma Linda U. Dept. Nutr., Personal Communication.

61. Colliers Encyclopedia, 15:607, 1969.
    Standard and Poor's Industry Reports, Vol.141(37):1, 1973.
    Bieler, H.G. Op.Cit., p. 123.
    Guthrie, H.A. "Introductory Nutrition," 2nd ed., p. 70, Mosby, 1971.
    Williams, R.J. "Nutrition Against Disease," p. 350, Bantam, 1971.
62. Azzopardi, J.G. and Whitticker, R.S.J. J.Clin.Path., 22:718, 1969.
    Lafferty, F.W. Medicine, 45:247, 1966.
    Glasko, G.S.B. and Burn, J.J. Brit.Med.J., 3:513, 1971.
    Benvenista, D.S., et al. Am.J.Med., 46:976, 1969.
    Muggia, F.M. and Heinemann, H.O. Ann.Inter.Med., 73:281, 1970.
    Stephens, R.L., et al. Cancer, 31:1487, 1973.
    Meyers, R. Arch.Surg., 80:308, 1960.
    Norris, L.C., et al. J.Nutr., 102:1085, 1972.
    Samaan, N.A. The Cancer Bulletin (U.Tex.at Houston), 25(5): 85, 1973.
    Davis, T.E., et al. Cornell Vet., 60:90, 1970.
    Krishnarao, G.V.G. and Draper, H.H. J.Nutr., 102:1143, 1972.
63. Ibid.
    Walker, R. and Linkswiler, H. J.Nutr., 102:1143, 1972.
    Johnson, N.E., et al. J.Nutr., 100(12):1425, 1970.
    Shah, B.G., et al. J.Nutr., 92(1):30, 1967.
    Hully, S.B., et al. J.Clin.Invest., 50(12):2506, 1971.
    Hammond, R.H. and Storey, E. Calf Tissue Res., 4(4):291, 1970.
    Odland, L.M., et al. Am.J.Clin.Nutr., 25:905, 1972.
    Ellis, F.R., Holish, S. and Ellis, J.W. Am.J.Clin.Nutr., 25:555, 1971.
64. Ibid.
    Davis, T.E., et al. Cornell Vet., 60:90, 1970.
    Krishnarao, G.V.G. and Draper H.H. J.Nutr., 102:1143, 1972.
    Johnson, N.E., et al. J.Nutr., 100(12):1425, 1970.
    Natenberg, M. Op.Cit., p. 143.
65. Bieler, H.G. Op.Cit., p. 199.
    Kelly, W.B. "New Hope for Cancer Victims," p. 23, The Kelly Research Foundation, 1969.
    Brandt, J. "The Grape Cure," Provoker Press (undated).
    Natenberg, M. Op.Cit., pp. 27, 43, 51, 75, 102.
66. Ross, M.H. and Bras, G. J.Nutr., 103(7):944, 1973.
67. Connell, H.C. Canad.M.A.J., 52:64, 1945.
    Tannenbaum, A. Cancer Res., 5(11):616, 1945; 9(3):162, 1949.

68. Hirayama, T. Op.Cit.
    Ishii, K., et al. Jap.J.Clin.Med., 26:1839, 1968.
    Wostmann, B.S. J. Nutr., 103(7):982, 1973.
    Bieler, H.G. Op.Cit., p. 21.
69. Anderson, D.E., et al. J.Natl.Cancer Inst., 45:697, 1970.
    Miller, D.S. and Parsonage, S.R. Proc.Soc.Nutr., 31:31A, 1972.
70. Anderson, D.E., et al. J.Natl.Cancer Inst., 45:497, 1970.
    Engel, R.W., et al. Ann.N.Y. Acad.Sci., 49:49, 1947.
    Okada, M. and Ochi, A. J.Biochem.(Japan), 70:581, 1971.
    Morris, H.P. Ann. N.Y.Acad.Sci., 49:119, 1947.
    Revlin, R.S. Cancer Res., 33(9): 1967, 1973.
71. Leuchtenberger, R., et al. Science, 101:46, 1945.
    Ibid. Proc.Soc.Exp.Bio.Med., 55:204, 1944.
    Greenblatt, M. J.Natl.Cancer Inst., 50:1055, 1973.
    Marjanen, H. and Soini, S. Agric.Fenn., 11(6):391, 1972.
72. Shamberger, R.J., et al. J.Natl.Cancer Inst., 50:863, 1973; 44: 931, 1970.
    Harr, J.R., et al. Clin.Toxicol., 5:187, 1972.
73. Burrell, R.J., et al. J.Natl.Cancer Inst., 36:201, 1966.
74. Krebs, E.T. and Bonziane, N.R. in "Control for Cancer," by Kittler, G.P. pp. 192–193, Warner, 1963.
75. Benet, Sula. Personal Communication.
    Schweitzer, A. Op.Cit.
    Haught, S.J. Op.Cit., p. 67.
    Bieler, H.G. Op.Cit., p. 218–230.
    Thomson, C.Leslie. The Kingston Chronicle, Edinburough, 1971.
    Natenberg, M. Op.Cit., p. 51.
    Tannenbaum, A. and Silverstone, H. Cancer Res., 13:460, 1953.
    Milker, D.M., et al. J.Nutr., 87:371, 1965.
    Arimatsu, Y. J.Kurume Med.Assn., 31:652, 1968.
    Frank, R.L. Am.J.Clin.Nutr., 22(4):464, 1969.
76. Steiner, P.E. Cancer Res., 2:425, 1942; 3:385, 1943; 7:273, 1947.
78. Burkholder, P.R. Science, June 18, 1943.
    Greenstein, J.P. Op.Cit., p. 248.
    McCance, R.A. and Widdowson, E.M. "The Composition of Foods," Her Maj.Stat.Office, 1960.
    Kamamoto, Y., et al. Cancer Res., 33(5):1129, 1973.
    Guthrie, H.A. Op.Cit., pp. 137–175.
    Hardinge, M.C. and Stare, E.J. J.Clin.Nutr., 2:73, 1954.
    Ellis, F.R. and Montejeffo, V.M.E. Plant Food Hum.Nutr., 2(2): 93, 1971.
    Ibid. Am.J.Clin.Nutr., 23:249, 1970.
    Banerjee, B. and Chakrabarti, C.H. J.Vitaminol., 16(3):235, 1970.

Hammond, R.H. and Strong, E. Calcif.Tissue Res., 4(4):291, 1970.

79. Marshall, M.W. and Hildebrand, H.E. J.Nutr., 19:227, 1963.
Chang, M.L.W., et al. J.Nutr., 101(3):323, 1971.
Markelova, V.F., et al. Byull.Eksp.Biol.Med., 69:50, 1970.

80. McCance, R.A. and Widdowson, E.M. Op.Cit., pp. 1868187.
Porter, J.W.G. and Rolls, B.A. Proc.Nutr. Soc., 30:17, 1971.
Uksila, E. and Kurkela, R. Maatal.Aikak., 38:221, 1966.
Kennaway, E.L. and Sampson, B.J. Pathol.Bactercol., 31:609, 1928.
Falk, H.L., et al. Cancer Res., 9:438, 1949.
Greenstein, J.P. Op.Cit., pp. 27–29, 1954.
Heiger, I. Brit.J.Cancer, 3:123, 1949.
Beck, S., et al. Cancer Res., 5:135, 1945.
Kirby, A.H.M. Cancer Res., 5:129, 1945.
Beinert, Frederica. Encyclopedia Americana, 7:749, 1971.
Bieler, H.G. Op.Cit., p. 190.

81. Schemmel, R., et al. J.Nutr., 100(9):1041, 1970.
Zaragoza, N. and Felber, J.P. Bio.Abs. 56119, 1971.
Akrens, R.A., et al. J.Nutr., 95(2):303, 1968.
Innami, M.G.Y., et al. Proc.Soc.Exptl.Bio.Med., 143:63, 1973.
Tremolieres, J., et al. Cah.Nutr.Diet., 5:37, 1970.
Velichko, A.A. Vopr.Pitan., 25(6):76, 1966.
Lemonnier, D., et al. Ann. Nutr.Aliment., 22:107, 1968.
DiCostanzo, G. Arch.Sci.Physiol., 24(1):337, 1970.
Schemmel, R., et al. J.Nutr., 102:1187, 1972.
Larsson, S. Acta Physiol.Scand., Suppl. 294, pp. 7–82, 1967.
Mayer, J. Postgrad Med., 43(6):205, 1968.
Miller, D.S. and Parsonage, S.R. Proc.Soc.Nutr., 31:31A, 1972.
McConnell, J.V. "Feedback, Fat and Freedom," Britannica Book of the Year, p. 35, Benton, 1973.
Fuge, K.W., et al. Am.J.Physiol., 214(3):660, 1968.
Canolazio, C.F. and Johnson, H.L. Am.J.Clin.Nutr., 25:85, 1972.
Lewis, S. and Guten, B. Am.J.Clin.Nutr., 26(9):1011, 1973.
Collnick, P.D., et al. J.Appl. Physiol., 33:421, 1972.
Leveille, G.A., et al. J.Nutr., 93:541, 1967.
Cohn, C. et al. Melab., 6:381, 1957.
Stevenson, J.A.F., et al. Proc.Soc.Exptl.Bio.Med., 116:178, 1964.
Leveille, G.A. and Hanson, R.W. Canad.J.of Physiol. and Pharmacology, 43:857, 1965.
Mukaida, C.S. and Lickton, I.J. J.Nutr., 101(6):767, 1971.
Leveille, G.A. J.Nutr., 91(2 pt 1):267, 1967.

Marshall, Mary, et al. Proc.Soc.Exptl.Bio. Med., 132(1):227, 1969.

Chaney, M.S. and Ross, M.L. "Nutrition" 7th Ed., p. 44, Haughton-Mifflen, 1966.

West, R.W. and Hayes, O.B. Am.J.Clin.Nutr., 21(8):853, 1968.

Groven, J.J. Am.J.Clin.Nutr., 20:191, 1967.

Hardinge, M.C. and Stare, F.J. J.Clin.Nutr., 2:73, 1954.

Ellis, R.F. and Montegriffo, V.M.E. Am.J.Clin.Nutr., 23:249, 1970.

Miller, D.S. and Rivers, J. Proc.Soc.Nutr., 31:32A, 1972.

Tremolieres, J., et al. Cah.Nutr.Diet 5:37, 1970.

82. Colliers Encyclopedia, 15:607, 1969.

86. Stump, D.J. Colliers Encyclopedia, 5:342, 1969.

Stein, J.J. Op.Cit.

87. Ibid.

Beinert, Frederica. Encyclopedia Americana, 7:749, 1971.

Encyclopedia Britannica, 4:769, 1969.

88. Price, W.A. Op.Cit.

Rotkin, J.D. Cancer Res., 33(6):1353, 1973.

Williams, R.J. Op.Cit., p. 141.

DeCastro, Josue. "The Geography of Hunger," Boston, Little, Brown, 1952.

89. Stump, D.J. Colliers Encyclopedia, 5:342, 1969.

Visscher, M.B., et al. Surgery, 11:48, 1942.

Sommers, S.C. Lab.Invest., 4:160, 1950.

Ibid., "Pathology Annual, Vol.8," Appleton, 1973.

Young, C.W., "The Americana Yearbook," p. 447, 1973.

Cancer News, 25(1):13, 1974.

90. Visscher, M.B., et al. Op.Cit.

Tannenbaum, Albert. Ann.N.Y. Acad.Science, 49:10, 1947.

Ross, M.H. Am.J.Clin.Nutr., 25:834, 1973.

91. Cancer News, 25(1):13, 1974.

Gammal, E.B., et al. Cancer Res., 27:1727, 1967; 28:384, 1968.

Carroll, K.K. and Khor, H.T. Cancer Res., 30:2260, 1970.

Ibid. Lipids, 6:415, 1971.

Stein, J.J. Op.Cit.

Chabon, A.B., et al. Op.Cit.

Buell, P. J.Natl.Cancer Inst., 51(5):1479, 1973.

Cancer News, 28(1):5, 1974.

Science, 101:46, 1945.

Loma Linda U.Adventist Health Study. "Summary of Results of Adventist Mortality Study," 1958–1965, received, 1974.

Drasar, B.S. and Irving, D. Brit.J.Cancer, 27(2):167, 1973.

Wynder, E.L., et al. Cancer, 13:559, 1960; 20:113, 1967.

Lea, A.J. Lancet, 2:332, 1966.

Carroll, K.K., et al. Can.Med.Assn.J., 98:590, 1968.

92. Price, W.A. Op.Cit.
    Loma Linda U., Op.Cit.
93a. Auerbach, O. and Sout, A. New Eng. J.Med., 295:253, 1961.
94. Wynder, E.L., et al. J.Natl.Cancer Inst., 51:391, 1973.
    Byrd, O.E. "Health" 3rd Ed., p. 202, Saunders, 1961.
    Diehl, H.S. and Dalrymple, W. "Healthful Living," p. 170, McGraw-Hill, 1968.
    Herber, L. Op.Cit., p. 147.
95. Benet, S. Personal Communication.
    Kurta, A.N. and Ellis, F.B. Plant Foods Hum.Nutr., 2(1):13, 1970.
    Personal interviews with vegans from London area, Spring, 1972.
    Grant, F., et al. Nutr.Abs.Rev. 4920,44(8):558, 1974.
96. Dean, G. Brit.Med.J., 2:852, 1959.
    Cornfield, J., et al. J.Natl.Cancer Inst., 22:176, 1959.
    Herber, L. Op.Cit., p. 149.
    Greenstein, J.P. Op.Cit., p. 28.
98. Cutler, S.J. Op.Cit.
    U.S. Dept. of Health, Education and Welfare, NIH, "end results of cancer," rep.no.4, p.5, 1972.
99. Cutler, S.J. Op.Cit.
100. Reddy, B.S. and Wynder, E.L. J.Natl.Cancer Inst., 50:1437, 1973.
    Hill, M.J., et al. Lancet, 1:95, 1970.
    Lacassagne, A., et al. Nature (U.K), 190:1007, 1961; 209:1026, 1966.
    Avigan, J. and Steinber, G.D. J.Clin.Invest., 44:1845, 1965.
101. Visscher, M.B., et al. Surgery, 11:48, 1942.
102. Haenszel, B., et al. J.Natl.Cancer Inst., 51(6):1765, 1973.
103. Visscher, M.B., et al. Surgery, 11:48, 1942.
    Berg, J.W. Lancet, p. 486, Sept. 2, 1972.
104. Drasar, B.S. and Hill, M.J. Am.J.Clin.Nutr., 25:1399, 1973.
    Newberne, P.M. and Rogers, A.E. J.Natl.Cancer Inst., 50:439, 1973.
    Roffo, A.H. Bol.Inst.Med.Exper.Estud. Trat.Cancer, 15:837, 1938.
105. Haught, S.J. Op.Cit., p. 67.
    MacDonald, E.J. The Cancer Bulletin, 25(2):40, 1973.
106. Cutler, S.J. Op.Cit.
    Pack, G.T. and Ariel, M. (eds) "Tumors of the Gastrointestinal Tract, Pancreas, Bilary System and Liver," 1962.
107. Abels, J.C., et al. Ann.Internal Med., 16:221, 1942.
108. Cutler, S.J. Op.Cit.
    Jones, H.W. Encyl.Amer., 22:670, 1971.
    Huggins, C. Physiol.Rev., 25:281, 1945.

110. Price, W.A. Op.Cit.
Larsson, S. Acta Physiol.Scand., Suppl.294, pp. 7–82, 1967.
Rosevear, R.F. Modern Nutrition, Nov.–Dec., 1964, Feb.–Mar., 1965.
Beauvoin, Simone de. "The Coming of Age," Putnum, 1972.

111. Cutler, S.J. Op.Cit.
U.S. Dept. of Health, Education and Welfare, NIH, "end results of cancer" rep. no. 4, p. 5, 1972.
Stein, J.J., Op.Cit.
Schmauz, R. and Cole, P.J. Natl.Cancer Inst., 52:1431, 1974.
Cole, P., et al. N.Eng.J.Med., 284, 129, 1971.
Ibid. Lancet, 1:1335, 1971.

112. Guthrie, H.A. Op.Cit., pp. 137–175.
Hardinge, M.C. and Stare, E.J. J. Clin.Nutr., 2:73, 1954.
Encyl.Brit., 4:596, 1969.
Nagy, M. J.Am.Med.Assoc., 226(8), Nov. 19, 1973.
Krishnarao, G.V.G. and Draper, H.H. J.Nutr., 102:1143, 1972.
Johnson, N.E., et al. J.Nutr., 100(12):1425, 1970.
Ross, M.H. and Bras, G. Op.Cit.

113. Cutler, S.J. Op.Cit.
U.S. Dept. of Health, Education and Welfare, NIH, "end results of cancer" rep. no. 4, p. 5, 1972.
Stump, D.J. Colliers Encyl., 5:344, 1969.
Mendel, M.A., et al. Cancer, 31:1408, 1973.
U.S. Pub.Health Service Pub. # 1103, 1964.
Staszewski, J. Brit.J.Cancer, 14:419, 1960; 23:247, 1969.
DuPlessis, L.S., et al. Nature, 222:1198, 1969.
Burrell, R.J., et al. Op.Cit.
Loma Linda U. Op.Cit.

114. Cutler, S.J. Op.Cit.
U.S. Dept. of Health, Education and Welfare, NIH, "end results of cancer," rep. no. 4, p. 5, 1972.
Encyl. Brit., 4:770, 1969.
Rains, A.J.H. Encyl. Amer., 12, 253, 1971.
Mitchell, et al. "Cooper's Nutrition in Health and Disease," 15th ed., Lippincott, 1968.
Bergman, F. Bio.Abs. 21392, 52:2237, 1971.
Berman, F., et al. Bio.Abs. 110415, 1967.
Dublin, L.I. "Factbook on Man," pp. 132, 145, 177, 301, McMillan, 1965.
Denbesten, L., et al. Op.Cit.
Miyake, H. and Johnston, C.G. Digestion, 1:219, 1968.
Nakayama, F. and Miyake, H. Am.J. Surg., 120:79, 1970.
Kameda, H. Gastroenterology, 46:109, 1964.

115. Hirayama, T. Op.Cit.
Ishii, K., et al. Jap.J.Clin.Med., 26:1839, 1968.
Singh, Inder. Lancet, 268:422, 1955.
Kessler, I.I. "Britannica Book of the Year," p. 473, 1971.
Ross, M.H. and Bras, G. Op.Cit.
116. Tannenbaum, A. Ann.N.Y.Acad.Sci. 49:9, 1947.
Kaunitz, H., et al. Z.Ernaehrungswiss, 10:61, 1970.
Rusch, H.P., et al. Cancer News, 5:431, 1945.
Lawrason, F.D. Proc.Soc.Exper.Biol.Med., 56:6, 1944.
Loma Linda U. Op.Cit.
117. Purtilo, D.T. and Gottlieb, L.S. Cancer, 32(8):458, 1973.
Encyl. Brit., 4:769, 1969.
Greenstein, J.P. Op.Cit., p. 248.
118. Silverstone, H. and Tannenbaum, A. Cancer Res., 11:443, 1951; 9:724, 1949.
Cancer Res., 9:162, 1949; 12:750, 1952.
120. Greenstein, J.P., Op.Cit., p. 509.
D'Ambrosio, J. Op.Cit.
Bieler, H.G. Op.Cit.
Haught, S.J. Op.Cit., p. 67.
Buckner, N. and Swaffield, M. Cancer Res., 33(12):3189, 1973.
121. Bieler, H.G. Op.Cit., pp. 20, 67, 68.
123. Brandt, J. Op.Cit., p. 44–45.
125. Haught, S.J. Op.Cit., p. 150.
U.S. Govt. Printing Office Document No. 89471.

References: Chapter II
137. Diehl, H.S. and Dalrymple, W. "Healthful Living," 8th ed., p. 37, McGraw-Hill, 1968.
Turner, R. and Ball, K. Lancet, p. 1137, Nov. 17, 1973.
Page, I. in "Your Heart," ed. by Montague, J.F., p. 94, Fawcett Publ., 1969.
138. Diehl, H.S. and Dalrymple, W. Op.Cit., p. 39.
Olsen, R.E. in "Life and Disease," ed. by Ingle, D.J., p. 211, Basic Books, 1963.
Robinson, C. "Proudfit-Robinson's Normal and Therapeutic Nutrition," 13th ed., p. 611, MacMillan, 1967.
Douglas, J.F. Annual Reports in Medicinal Chemistry, 78:180, 1969.
142. Olsen, R.E., Op.Cit.
Robinson, C. Op.Cit.
Douglas, J.F. Op.Cit.
St.Clair, R.W., et al. Exp. Mol.Pathol., 15(1):21, 1971.

Gutierrez, S.M. An.Fac.Quim.Farm, 18:133, 1966.

Talbott, G.D., et al. Ann.Inter.Med., 54:257, 1961.

Olsen, R.E. Op.Cit., p. 234.

144. Enos, W.F., et al. J.A.M.A., 152:1090, 1953.

Herber, L. "Our Synthetic Environment," p. 8, Knopf, 1962.

Gubner, R. in "Your Heart" ed. by Montague, J.F. p. 111, Fawcett, 1969.

Pesonen, E. Athero., 20:173, 1974.

145. Blakeslee, A. and Stamler, J. "Your Heart Has Nine Lives," pp. 15, 50–51, Prentice-Hall, 1963.

Groen, J.J. Am.J.Clin.Nutr., 20:191, 1967.

Herber, L. Op.Cit., p. 15.

Baldry, P.E. "The Battle Against Heart Disease," pp. 123–4, Cambridge U.Press, 1971.

Loma Linda U. "Adventist Health Study," 1974.

146. Benet, S. "Abkhasians," p. 12, Holt, Rinehart and Winston, 1974.

Leaf, A. Ntl.Geo., 143(1):93, 1973.

Armstrong, T. Soil and Health J. (N.Z.), Oct–Nov, 1965.

147. Herber, L. Op.Cit., p. 8.

Benet, S. N.Y.Times, Dec. 26, 1971.

148. Sabbaugh, M.E. Assoc.Prof., Geogr., U.Tex., Personal Communication.

149. Blakeslee, A. and Stamler, J. Op.Cit., p. 47.

Turner, R. and Ball, K. Op.Cit.

Editorial. "Diet and Coronary Heart Disease," Am.J.Clin.Nutr., 26:53, 1973.

Burn, H. "Our Most Interesting Diseases," p. 114, Scribner's Sons, 1964.

White, P. in "Your Heart" Op.Cit., p. 27.

Kloppers, P.J. Afr.J.Med.Sci., 2(4):387, 1971.

150. Samuel, P., et al. Am.J.Clin.Nutr., 23:178, 1970.

Yudkin, J. "Sucrose in the Aetiology of Cor.Thromb. and Other Diseases," Butterworths, 1971.

Blakeslee, A. and Stamler, J. Op.Cit., p. 48.

Boylan, B.R. "The New Heart," pp. 157–160, Chilton, 1969.

Allard, Claude and Goulet, Claude. Can.Med.Assn.J., 98(13): 627, 1968.

Wertlake, P.T. New Physician, 8:41, 1959.

Blakeslee, A. and Stamler, J. Op.Cit., p. 48.

151. Editorial. "Diet and Coronary Heart Disease," Op.Cit.

152. Ellis, R.F. and Montegriffo, V.M.E. Am.J.Clin.Nutr., 23:249, 1970.
Walker, G.R., et al. J.Nutr., 72:317, 1960.
Kask, E. Exp.Med.Surg., 27(3):290, 1969.
Hodges, R.E., et al. Am.J.Clin.Nutr., 20:198, 1967.
Ellis, F.R. and Montegriffo, V.M.E. Plant Foods Hum.Nutr. 2(2): 93, 1971.
153. Hardinge, M.C. and Stare, F.J. J.Clin.Nutr., 2:73, 1954; 2:83, 1954.
West, R.O. and Hayes, O.B. Am.J.Clin.Nutr., 21(8):853, 1968.
Kirkley, K. Acta Med. Scand., 180(6):767, 1966.
154. Rickman, F., et al. J.A.M.A., 228(1):54, 1974.
158. Quintão, E., et al. J.Lipid Res., 12(2):233, 1971.
Mattson, F.H., et al. Am.J.Clin.Nutr., 25:589, 1972.
Hegested, D.M., et al. Am.J.Clin.Nutr., 17:281, 1965.
159. Mattson, F.H., et al. Op.Cit.
160. Ibid.
Hegested, D.M., et al. Op.Cit.
161. Gosling, R.G., et al. J.Athero., 9(1):47, 1969.
Splitter, S.D., et al. Metab. (Clin.Exp.), 17(12):1129, 1968.
Fisher, H. N.J.Agr.Exp.Sta.Coll.Agr.Environ.Sci.Bull. 819, pp. 3–7, 1968.
Robinson, C. Op.Cit., p. 613.
Arvidson, G. and Halmros, H. Z.Ernaerungswiss, 11:105, 1972.
Newman, W.P. III, et al. Athero., 19:75, 1974.
162. Armstrong, M.L. and Megan, M.B. Circ.Res., 30:675, 1972.
163. Malmros, H., et al. Acta Med.Scand., 192:201, 1972.
Lindall, A.W., et al. Proc.Soc.Exp.Biol.Med., 136(9):1032, 1971.
Maguire, K.F. and Doran, G.A. Am.J.Anat., 135:153, 1972.
Rozynknowa, D., et al. Op.Cit.
164. Connor, W.E., et al. J.Clin.Invest., 48(8):1363, 1969.
Steinbach, M., et al. Rev.Roum.Med.Intern., 5:103, 1968.
Goldsmith, G.A., et al. Bull.Tulane U. Med.Fac., 27(1):1, 1968.
Malmros, R. and Wigand, G. Lancet, 2:1, 1957.
165. Kaunitz, H., et al. Z.Ernaehrungswiss, 10(1):61, 1970.
Pawar, S.S. and Tidwell, H.C. Am.J.Physiol., 213(6):1358, 1967.
Hanson, D., et al. Am.J.Physiol., 213:(2):347, 1967.
Howard, A.N. and Gresham, G.A. Int.Z.Vitaminforsch., 38: 545, 1968.
Fraham, H., et al. Milchwissenschaft, 22:206, 1967.
Karvonen, M.J. Proc.Nutr., Soc., 31:355, 1972.
Evans, D.W., et al. Lancet, 2:172, 1972.
Brerenbaum, M.L., et al. J.A.M.A., 202:1119, 1967.

166. Howard, A.N. and Gresham, G.A. Op.Cit.
167. Trowell, H. Am.J.Clin.Nutr., 25:926, 1972.
168. Eatwood, M. Lancet, Dec. 6, 1969.
     DeGroot, A.P., et al., Lancet, 2:303, 1963.
     Mathur, K.S., et al. Brit.Med.J., 1:30, 1968.
169. Kritchevsky, D., et al. J.Athero.Res., 8(4):697, 1968.
     Fisher, H. and Grimenger, P., Proc.Soc.Exptl.Biol.Med., 126:108, 1967.
     Shafrir, E., et al. Isr.J.Med.Sci., 8:990, 1972.
     Carroll, K. K. Atherosclerosis, 13:(1):67, 1971.
     Trowell, H. Op.Cit.
     Cookson, F.B., et al. J.Athero. Res., 7:69, 1967.
     More, J.H. Brit.J.Nutr., 21:207, 1967.
     Devi, K.S. and Karup, P.A. Athero., 11:479, 1970.
     Vyayagopalan, P. and Karup, P.A. Athero., 11:257, 1970; 15:215, 1972.
     Kitchevsky, D. and Tepper, S.A. J.Athero.Res., 8:357, 1968.
     Balmer, J. and Zilversmit, D.B. J.Nutr., 104:1319, 1974.
170. Eastwood, M. Lancet, Dec. 6, p. 222, 1969.
     Chakrabarti, C.H. Indian J.Exp.Bio., 5(4):222, 1967.
     Portman, O.W. and Murphy, P. Arch.Biochem.Biophys., 76:367, 1958.
171. Bruckdorfer, K.R., et al. Nutr.Metab., 13(1):36, 1971.
     Khan, I.H. and Yadkin, J. Proc.Nutr.Soc., 30:74A, 1971.
     Schroeder, M. J.Nutr., 97:237, 1969.
     Staub, H.W. and Ghressen, R. J.Nutr., 95(4):633, 1968.
     Nakai, T. Jap.Circ.J., 35(4):465, 1971.
     Chunakova, E.P., Ter.Arkh., 43:78, 1971.
172. Olsen, R.E. Op.Cit., pp. 232–236.
     Akinyanju, P. and Yudkin, J. Nature, 214(5086):426, 1967.
     Naismith, D.J., et al. J.Nutr., 97(3):375, 1969.
173. Chunakova, E.P., et al. Sov.Med., 30(8):30, 1967.
     Kiriyama, S., et al. J.Nutr., 97(3):382, 1969.
     Williams, R.J. "Nutrition Against Disease," pp. 293–294, Bantam Books, 1973.
175. Boechko, F.F. Vopr.Pitan., 30(4):21, 1971.
     Hamuro, Y. J.Nutr., 101(5):635, 1971.
     Schroeder, H.A. Am.J.Clin.Nutr., 21(3):230, 1968.
     Weber, C.E. J.Theor.Biol., 29(2):327, 1970.
176. Ellis, R.F. and Montegriffo, V.M.E. Am.J.Clin.Nutr., 23:249, 1970.
     Ringer, R.K., et al. Poult.Sci., 51(3):925, 1972.
     Kordylas, J.M. Lancet, Sept. 16, p. 606, 1972.
     Ginter, E., et al. Nutr.Metab., 12(2):76, 1970.
     Williams, R.J., Op.Cit., pp. 78–79.
     Kopjas, T., J.Am.Geriac.Soc., 14:1187, 1966.

Parsons, W.B. in "Your Heart," Op.Cit., p. 69.

Banerjee, B. and Chakrabart, C.H. J.Nutr.Diet., 3(3):72, 1966.

Kaneda, T. and Tokuda, S. J.Nutr., 90(4):371, 1966.

178. Blakeslee, A. and Stamler, J. Op.Cit., p. 56.

Havel, R.J. and Carlson, L.A. Metab., 11:195, 1962.

Moses, C. "Atherosclerosis," p. 153, Lea and Febiger, 1963.

179. Ibid, p. 132.

Havel, R.J. and Carlson, L.A. Op.Cit.

Allard, Claude and Goulet, Claude. Op.Cit.

180. Edwards, C.H., et al. Am.J.Clin.Nutr., 24(2):181, 1971.

Hodges, R.E., et al. Am.J.Clin.Nutr., 20:198, 1967.

Kirkley, K. Acta Med.Scand., 180:767, 1966.

181. Kritchevsky, D., et al. J.Ather.Res., 8(4):697, 1968.

Bruckdorfer, K.R., et al. Nutr., Metab., 13(1):36, 1971.

Ibid., Proc.of Nutr.Soc., 31:11A, 1972.

Gontea, I., et al. Fiziol. Norm. Patol., 16(5):403, 1970.

Bruckdorfer, K.R., et al. Biochem J., 129: 439, 1972.

Lang, C.M. and Barthel, C.H. Am.J.Clin.Nutr., 25(1972).

Jourdan, M.H. Nutr.Metab., 14:28, 1972.

Chevalier, M., et al. Proc.Soc.Exp.Bio.Med., 139(1):220, 1972.

Naismith, D.H. and Khan, N.A. Proc.Nutr.Soc., 29:64A, 1970.

Bruckdorfer, K.R. Proc.Soc.Nutr., 30:74A, 1971.

182. Hulley, S.B., et al. Lancet, Sept. 16, 1972.

Grande, F., et al. Am.J.Clin.Nutr., 25(1):53, 1972.

Wadhwa, P., et al. Am.J.Clin.Nutr., 26(8):823, 1973.

Mann, J.I. and Truswell, A.S. Br.J.Nutr., 27(2):395, 1972.

Anderson, J.T. Am.J.Clin.Nutr., 20:168, 1967.

Friedman, M., et al. Proc.Soc.Exp.Biol.Med., 135(3):785, 1970.

Kaufmann, N.A., et al. Am.J.Clin.Nutr., 18:261, 1966.

Am.J.Clin.Nutr., 20:131, 1967.

Bosch, V., et al. Acta Cient.Venez., 18(2):50, 1967.

183. Kuo, P.T., et al. Am.J.Clin.Nutr., 20:116, 1967.

184. Kritchevsky, D., et al. Op.Cit.

McGregor, D. Br.J.Nutr., 25(2):213, 1971.

Cheraskin, E. and Ringsdorf, W.M. J.Oral.Med., 23(3/4):124, 1969.

185. Little, J.A., et al. Atherosclerosis, 11(2):173, 1970.

Antar, M.A., et al. Atherosclerosis, 11(2):191, 1970.

Albrink, M.J. and Meigs, J.W. Am.J.Clin.Nutr., 24:344, 1971.

Lopez, A., et al. Gerontol.Clin., 13:171, 1971.

McDonald, I. Proc.Nutr.Soc., 30:72A, 1971.

Birchwood, B.L., et al. Ather., 11:183, 1970.

Mann, J.I., et al. Clin. Sci. (Oxford), 44(6):601, 1973.

Wilson, S.W., et al. Am.J.Med., 51:491, 1971.

Rickman, F., et al. J.A.M.A., 227:54, 1974.

187. Karvonen, M.J. Proc.Nutr.Soc., 31:355, 1972.
Chunakova, E.P. Op.Cit.
Wilson, S.W., et al. Op.Cit.

188. Yudkin, J. "Sweet and Dangerous," pp. 94–96, Bantam Books, 1972.

190. Olsen, R.E. Op.Cit., pp. 213, 221.
Tong, P. Nat.Obs., Nov. 23, 1974.
Chang, M.W., et al. J.Nutr., 96(3):368, 1968.
Marshall, M.W. and Hildebrand, H.E. J.Nutr., 19:227, 1963.
Varnell, T.R. and Chang, Y.-O. Biochem.Biophys.Acta, 266(2): 444, 1972.
Taylor, D.D., et al. J.Nutr., 91:275, 1967.
Chalvardjian, A. J.Nutr., 101(2):193, 1971.
Chalvardjian, A. and Stephens, S. J.Nutr., 100(4):397, 1970.
Nakamura, T., et al. Tohoku J.Exp.Med., 93(3):227, 1967.
Chang, M.L.W., et al. J.Nutr. 101(3):323, 1971.

192. Beevers, D.G., et al. Lancet, p. 1407, June 23, 1973.
Blakeslee, A. and Stamler, J. Op.Cit., p. 143.

193. Burn, H. Op.Cit., pp. 91–92.
Davidson, S., Meikelejohn, A.P. and Passmore, R. "Human Nutrition and Dietitics," p. 555, Williams and Wilkins, 1961.
Burn, H. Op.Cit., p. 93.

194. Gubner, R. in "Your Heart," Op.Cit., p. 110.
Davidson, S., Meikelejohn, A.P. and Passmore, R. Op.Cit., pp. 555–556.
Whyte, H.M. Aust.Ann.Med., 7:36, 1958.

195. Davidson, S., Miekelejohn, A.P. and Passmore, R. Op.Cit, pp. 555–556.
Hanssen, M. "About the Salt of Life," pp. 15, 16, 23, 24, 25, Thorsons, 1968.
Bieler, H.G. "Food is Your Best Medicine," pp. 219–220, Vintage, 1973.
Master, A.M., Garfield, C.L. and Walters, M.B. "Normal Blood Pressure and Hypertension," p. 63, Lea and Febiger, 1952.
Pasricha, S. J.Nutr.Diet., 3(3):79, 1966.
Chaney, M.S. and Ross, M.L. "Nutrition," 7th ed., pp. 180–181, Houghton-Mifflin, 1966.

196. Karl, R.M. in "Modern Nutrition in Health and Disease," 3rd ed., p. 851, ed by. Wohl, M.G. and Goodhart, R.S., Lea and Febiger, 1964.
Page, I.H., McCubbin, J.W. and Corcoran, A.C., in "Life and Disease," ed. by Ingle, D.J., Basic Books, 1963.
Pickering, G.W. "The Nature of Essential Hypertension," p. 117, Grune and Stratton, 1961.

197. Bieler, H.G. Op.Cit., pp. 136–137.
198. Hanssen, M. Op.Cit. pp. 23–24.
    Schackow, E. and Dahl, L.K. Proc.Soc.Exptl.Bio.and Med., 122: 952, 1966.
    Jaffe, D., et al. Arch.Pathol., 90(1):1, 1970.
    Arimatsu, Y. J.Kurume Med.Assn., 31(7):652, 1968.
    Fapeeva, V.K. Gig.Saint., 36:11, 1971.
    Fugii, J., et al. Tohoku, J.Exp.Med., 97(3):191, 1969.
    Lenel, R., et al. Am.J.of Physiol., 152:557, 1948.
    Menard, J., et al. Pathol.Biol., 19:821, 1971.
    Gavras, H., et al. Clin.Sci., 38(4):409, 1970.
199. Trangeizer, V.A., et al. Vopr.Pitan., 30(4):32, 1971.
    Dahl, L.K. and Love, R.A. Proc.Fed. of Am.Soc.for Exptl.Bio., 15: 513, 1956.
    Zusmanovich, V.A. Sov.Med., 32(2):138, 1969.
200. Talbott, G.D., et al. Ann.Inter.Med., 54:257, 1961.
203. Price, J.M. "Coronaries-Cholesterol-Chlorine," pp. 65–69, Pyramid, 1971.
    Hopkins, E.S. "Water Purification Control," Williams and Wilkins, 1948.
204. Burstyn, P.G., et al. Br.J.Exp.Pathol., 53:258, 1972.
    Douglas, B.H. and Langford, H.G. Clin.Res., 17:83, 1969.
    Arai, K. Tohoku Igaku Zasshi, 82(5):246, 1970.
    Elin, R.J., et al. Am.J.Physiol., 220(3):543, 1971.
    Mikhel'son, D.A. Vopr.Pitan., 28(6):54, 1969.
    Oomen, H.A.P.C. Voeding, 28(1):3, 1967.
205. Kasper, H. and Kuehn, H.A. Med.Ernahr., 11:52, 1970.
    Aoyama, G., et al. J.Nutr., 97(3):348, 1969.
    Krylova, E.A. Urol. Nefrol., 33(3):18, 1968.
    Polec, R., et al. Pol.Arch.Med.Wewn., 40(4):449, 1968.
    Pronchenko, I.A. Klin.Med., 46(1):51, 1968.
    Dolgodvorow, A.F., et al. Ter.Arkh., 41(1):93, 1969.
    Tareev, E.M., et al. Vopr.Pitan., 31(2):8, 1972.
207. Kempner, W. North Carolina M.J. 5:125, 273; 6:62, 117, 1944–45.
    Mitchell, H.S., et al. "Cooper's Nutr. in Health and Disease," 15th Ed., Lippincott, p. 341, 1968.
    Meyer, B.J., et al. S.Africa Medical Journal, 45(8):191, 1971.
    Chase, A. "Nutrition for Health," pp. 71–73, Parker, 1954.
208. Master, A.M., Garfield, C.L. and Walters, M.B. "Normal Blood Pressure and Hypertension," p. 63, Lea and Febiger, 1952.
211. Yudkin, J. "Sucrose in the Aetiology of Cor.Thromb. and Other Diseases," Butterworths, 1971.

212. Boylan, B.R. "The New Heart," Chilton, 1969.
Dudenko, N.V. Vopr.Okhr.Materin.Det., 14(9):83, 1969.
Balestreri, R. and Bertolini, S. Arch.Marag.Patol.Clin., 27:45, 1971.
Lesnichii, A.V. Vopr.Pitan., 27(2):86, 1968.
Shepard, W.W., et al. Modern Medicine, Dec. 1, 1960.
Szent-Gyorgyi, N. Am.J.Clin.Nutr., 5:244, 1957.

215. English, J.P. et al. J.A.M.A., 115:1327, 1940.
Mills, C.A. and Porter, M.M. Am.J.Med.Sci., 234:35, 1957.
Hammond, E.C. Am.J.Public Health, 50:20, 1960.

216. Boylon, B.R. Op.Cit., pp. 157–160.
U.S. Dept. of H.E.W. "Smoking and Health," p. 325, D.Van Nostrand, undated.
Poole, L. "I Am A Chronic Cardiac," Dodd Mead, p. 6, 1969.

217. Benet, S. "Abkhasians," p. 25, Holt, Rinehart and Winston, 1974.
Ellis, R.F. and Montegriffo, V.M.E. Am.J.Clin.Nutr., 23:249, 1970. Auerbach, S. Op.Cit.

218. Richardson, J.F. Br.J.Nutr., 27(3):449, 1972.
Med.Research Council Working Party. Lancet, 2(7686):1265, 1970.

219. Baldry, P.E. "The Battle Against Heart Disease," Cambridge U.Press, 1971.
White, P.D. in "Your Heart," Op.Cit., p. 17.
Burn, A. Op.Cit., pp. 114–115.

220. The Wall Street Journal. April 2, 1974.
Link, R.P. Athero., 15:107, 1972.
Rochelle, R. Res.Quar. Am.Assn.Health Phys.Ed., 32:538, 1961.
Lopez, S.A., et al. Athero., 20:1, 1974.

222. Lingston, G.E., et al. Fd.Tech., 28:16, 1974.

224. Ibid.

231. Karvonen, M.J. Proc.Nutr.Soc., 31:355, 1972.
Blakeslee, A. and Stamler, J. Op.Cit., pp. 67–69.

232. Karvonen, M.J. Proc.Nutr.Soc., 31:355, 1972.

233. Blakeslee, A. and Stamler, J.S. Op.Cit, pp. 67–69.

234. Karvonen, M.J. Proc.Nutr.Soc., 31:355, 1972.
Blakeslee, A. and Stamler, J. Op.Cit., pp. 67–69.

235. Auerbach, S. Austin Am.Statesman, Nov. 29, 1974.

References: Chapter III

251. Lubin, J.S. Wall Street J., Nov. 4, 1974.
     Keene, H. Proc.Nutr. Soc., 31:339, 1972.
252. Lubin, J.S. Op.Cit.
253. Ibid.
     Oshovskaya-Tsaifir, T.F., et al. Circ., 50:10, 1974.
254. Yudkin, J. "Sweet and Dangerous," Bantam Books, 1972.
255. Ibid.
     Bender, A.E. and Thandani, P.V. Nutr.Metab., 12(1):22, 1970.
     Cohen, A.M., et al. Am.J.Ophthalmol., 73:863, 1972.
     Rosenmann, E., et al. Diabetes, 20(12):803, 1971.
     Schroeder, H.A., et al. J.Nutr., 101(2):247, 1971.
256. Cohen, A.M. and Teitelbaum, A. Am.J.Physiol., 206:105, 1964.
     Dunnigan, M.G. Clin.Sci. (London), 38(1):1, 1970.
257. Matsuo, T., et al. Endocrinol. Jap., 17(6):477, 1970.
     Keene, H. Op.Cit.
258. Brunzell, J.D., et al. New Eng. J.Med., 284:521, 1971.
     Anderson, J.W., et al. Am.J.Clin.Nutr., 26:600, 1973.
     Yudkin, J. Proc.Nutr.Soc., 31:331, 1972.
     Parra, A. et al. Pediatric Res., 5(11):605, 1971.
     Goldrick, R.B., et al. Metab. Clin.Exp., 21:761, 1972.
     Taeufel, K. and Taeufel, A. Nahrung., 15(2):191, 1971.
     Yudkin, J. Op.Cit.
259. Robinson, C.H. "Proudfit-Robinson's Normal and Therapeutic Nutrition," 13th ed., pp. 564–572, MacMillan, 1967.
     Hausmann, T., et al. Nutr. Rev., 44:402, 1974.
     Katsumata, K. Nagoya J.Med.Sci., 32(2):261, 1970; 33(1):27, 1970.
260. Bourdel, G. Arch.Sci.Physio., 21(1):1, 1967.
     Berdanier, C.D. and Marshall, M.W. Nutr.Rep.Int., 3(6):383, 1971.
     Hodges, R.E. Nutr.Rev., 24:257, 1966.
     Keene, H. Op.Cit.
     Bieler, H.G. "Food is Your Best Medicine," Vintage, 1973.
     Chase, A. "Nutrition for Health," Parker, 1954.
     Robinson, C.H. Op.Cit.
263. Singh, I. Lancet, 268:422, 1955.
265. Kapadia, Rojesh. Personal Communication, March 19, 1975.
268. Dudenko, N.V. Vop.Okhr.Materin.Det., 14(9):83, 1969.
     Baletreri, R. and Bertolini, S. Arch.Marg.Patol.Clin., 27(2):45, 1971.
     Lesnichii, A.V. Vop.Pitan., 27(2):86, 1968.
     Dublin, L.I. "Factbook on Man," 2nd ed., pp. 132, 145, 177, 301, MacMillan, 1965.
269. Salans, L.B., et al. J.Clin.Inv., 52:929, 1973.

Bjorntorp, P. and Sjostrom, L. Metab.Clin.Exp., 20:703, 1971.
270. Guenther, S. Med.Welt., 6:386, 1968.
Marks, H.H. Metab., 6:417, 1957.
Ross, M.H. Am.J.Clin.Nutr., 25:834, 1972.
Young, P. Natl.Obs., Nov. 16, 1974.
271. Ibid.
Cheraskin, E. and Ringsdorf, W.M. "New Hope for Incurable Diseases," pp. 7–8, Arco, 1971.
Wiedorowicz, H. and Sterkowicz, S. Pol.Arch.Med.Wewn., 29, 287, 1967.
Mohr, M. Z.Gesamte. Inn.Med.Grenz., 24:907, 1969.
272. Miller, D.S. and Rivers, J. Proc.Soc.Nutr., 31:32A, 1972.
Benet, S. New York Times, December 26, 1971.
273. Ibid.
Kask, E. Exp.Med.Surg., 27(3):290, 1969.
Mardinge, M.C. and Stare, F.J. J.Clin.Nutr., 2:73, 1954; 2:83, 1954.
Ellis, R.F. and Montegriffo, V.M.E. Am.J.Clin.Nutr., 23:249, 1970.
Meyer, B.J., et al. S.Africa. Medical Journal, 45(8):191, 1971.
Cetera, N.E. Idia, 241:6, 1968.
274. Bieler, H.G. Op.Cit., p. 147.
Chase, A. Op.Cit., pp. 135–136.
276. Trangeizer, V.A., et al. Vop.Pitan., 30(4):32, 1971.
West, R.O. and Hayes, O.B. Am.J.Clin.Nutr., 21:853, 1968.
278. Alling, C. J.Nutr., 102(6):773, 1972.
DiCostanzo, G. Arch.Sci.Physiol., 24:337, 1970.
Zaragoza, N. and Felber, J.P. Horm.Metab.Res., 2(6):323, 1970.
Lemonnier, D. Nutr.Dieta, 9(1):27, 1967.
Prichard, R.W., et al. Arch.Pathol., 85(2):204, 1968.
Velichko, A.A. Vop.Pitan., 25(6):76, 1966.
279. Tremolieres, J., et al. Cah.Nutr.Diet., 5(1):37, 1970.
Naismith, D.J., et al. Proc.Soc.Nutr., 31:94A, 1972.
Larsson, S. Acta Physiol.Scand., Suppl. 294, pp. 7–82, 1967.
280. Mikelsen, Olaf, et al. J.Nutr., 57:541, 1971.
Miller, D.S. and Parsonage, S.R. Proc.Nutr.Soc., 31:31A, 1972.
U.S.Dept.Agr. "Composition of Foods," Handbook #8, pp. 13, 18, Revised, 1963.
281. Stein, J.M., et al. Metab.Clin.Exp., 20(10):903, 1971.
Sack, M.J. Proc.Nutr.Soc., 31:15A, 1971.
Miller, D.S. and Parsonage, S.R. Proc.Nutr.Soc., 31:31A, 1972.
282. Lemonnier, D., et al. Nutr.Metab., 16:15, 1974.
Markuske, H. Arztl.Jugendk., 60:296, 1969.
Bloom, W.L. and Eidex, M.F. Metabol.Clin.Exp., 16(8):679, 1967.
McConnell, J.V., "Brit. Book Yr.", p. 35, Benton, 1973.

283. Chittenden, R.H. "Physiological Economy in Nutrition," Stokes, 1904.

Pettenkofer, M. and Voit, C. Z.Biol., 2, 1866.

Chaney, M.S. and Ross, M.L. "Nutrition," 7th Ed., pp. 104–105, Houghton Mifflin, 1966.

Astand, P.O. Fed.Proc., 26(6):1772, 1967.

Hedman, R. Acta Physiol.Scand., 40:305, 1957.

Canolazio, C.F. and Johnson, H.L. Am.J.Clin.Nutr., 25:85, 1972.

Bergstrom, J., et al. Acta Physiol.Scand., 71:140, 1967.

Karlsson, J. and Saltin, B. J.Appl.Physiol., 3:203, 1971.

Kvartovkina, L.K. and Minkh, A.A. Gig.Sanit., 33(3):75, 1968.

Christensen, E.H. "Das Essen und Trinken des Sportlers. Sportmedizinsche Schuftenreihe," Bern: Wanderer, 1958.

Fuge, K.W., et al. Am.J.Physiol., 215(3):660, 1968.

Barboriak, J.J. and Wilson, A.S. J.Nutr., 102:1543, 1972.

Ahrens, R.A. and Wilson, J.E. J.Nutr., 90(1):63, 1966.

Henhede, M. "Protein and Nutrition," Ewart, Seymour, 1913.

285. Barboriak, J.J. and Wilson, A.S. J.Nutr., 103:1543, 1972.

Ahrens, R. and Wilson, J.E. J.Nutr., 90(1):63, 1966.

286. Swank, R.L. "A Biological Basis for Multiple Sclerosis," pp. 38–52, Thomas, 1961.

Swank, R.L. Arch.Neurol., 23:466, 1970.

Swank, R.L. and Grimsgaard, A. "Low-fat Diet; Reasons, Rules, and Recipes," U.Oregon, 1959.

287. Kempner, W. N.Car.Med.J., 5:125, 1944.

Watkin, D.M., et al. Am.J.Med., 9:428, 1950.

Chapman, C.B. N.E.J.Med., 243:899, 1950.

Currens, J.H., et al. N.E.J.Med., 245:354, 1951.

Dole, V.P., et al. J.Clin.Invest., 29:1187, 1950.

Page, I.H. and Corcoran, A.C. J. Clin.Nutr., 1:7, 1952.

Dole, V.P., et al. Am.J.Clin.Nutr., 2(6):381, 1954.

Williamson, C.R., New Eng.J.Med., 243:177, 1950.

288. Anand, C. and Linkwiler, H. J.Nutr., 104:695, 1974.

Ruckman, F., et al. J.A.M.A., 228(1):54, 1974.

289. Thomson, T.J. Lancet, 7471:992, 1966.

Ball, M.F., et al. J.Clin.Endocrinol.Metab., 27(2):273, 1967.

Graczykowska-Koczorowska, A., et al. Z.Ernaehrungswiss, 11:1, 1972.

Bruch, H. "The Importance of Overweight," p. 348, Norton, 1957.

Zuliani, U., et al. Ateneo.Parmen.Sez.1 Bio-Med., 40(6):549, 1969.

291. Schemmel, R., et al. J.Nutr., 102:1187, 1972.

292. Marshall, M., et al. Proc.Soc.Exp.Bio.Med., 132(1):227, 1969.

Mickelsen, O., et al. J.Nutr., 57:541, 1955.

Naismith, D.J., et al. Proc.Nutr.Soc., 29:56A, 1970.
293. Cabanae, M. and Duclaux, R. Science (Wash.), 168(3930):496, 1970.
Yudkin, J. Op.Cit.
296. Pawan, G.L.S. Proc.Soc.Nutr., 31:90A, 1972.
Dawidowicz, A. Wiad.Lek., 24:1623, 1971.
Cohn, C. and Joseph, D. Am.J.Phys., 196:965, 1959.
Tevin, L. Am.J.Physiology, 141:143, 1944.
Cohn, C. and Joseph, D. J.Nutr., 96(1):94, 1968.
Wardlaw, J.M., et al. Can.J.Physiol.Pharmacol., 47(1):47, 1969.
Cohn, C., et al. Metabolism, 6:381, 1957.
Padwaldesai, S.R. Br.J.Nutr., 23(4):745, 1969.
Stevenson, J.A.F., et al. Proc.Soc.Exp.Biol.Med., 116:178, 1964.
Leveille, G.A. and Hanson, R.W. Canadian J. of Physiology and Pharmacology, 43:857, 1965.
Mukaida, C.S. and Lichton, I.J. J.Nutr., 101(6):767, 1971.
Patel, M.S. and Mistry, S.P. J.Nutr., 97(4):496, 1969.
Alee, G.L., et al. J.Nutr., 102:1115, 1972.
Leveille, G. and O'Hea, E.K. J.Nutr., 93:541, 1967.
Romsos, D.R. Proc.Soc.Exp.Bio.Med., 139:868, 1972.
Leveille, G.A. and Hanson, R.W. Journal of Lipid Research, 7:46, 1966.
Leveille, G.A. J.Nutr., 91(2 part 1):267, 1967; 102(4):549, 1972.
Okey, R. J.Am.Diet.Assoc., 36:441, 1960.
297. Parsons, W.B. in "Your Heart," Op.Cit. p. 69.
Sydorenko, O.I. Pediatr.Akush.Ginekol., 32:12, 1970.
298. Pawan, G.L.S. Proc.Soc.Nutr., 31:90A, 1972.
299. Yudkin, J. "Sweet and Dangerous," pp. 122, 123, 134, Bantam Books, 1973.
Anderson, J.W., et al. Am.J.Clin.Nutr., 26:660, 1973.
300. Abrahamson, E.M. and Pezet, A.W. "Body, Mind and Sugar," pp. 177–182, 221–22, Pyramid, 1961.
302. Ibid.
303. Yudkin, J. "Sweet and Dangerous," Op.Cit., pp. 121–122.
304. Abrahamson, E.M. and Pezet, A.W. Op.Cit., pp. 219–220.
309. Schindler, J.A. Reader's Digest, Dec., 1949.
Price, W.A. "Nutrition and Physical Degeneration," Am.Acad.Nutr., 1950.
310. Abrahamson, E.M. and Pezet, A.W., Op.Cit., pp. 205–216.
311. Watson, G. "Nutrition and Your Mind," Bantam, 1972.
316. Wolbach, S.B. in "The Vitamins," Vol. I, ed. by Sebrell, W.H. and Harris, R.S., pp. 119–121, Academic Press, 1954.
Lillie, R.D. Natl.Inst.Health.Bull., 162:13, 1933.
Jensenius, H.; Norgaard, F. Acta.Pathol.Microbio.Scand., 19:433, 1942.
Hundley, J.M. in "The Vitamins," Vol. III, Op.Cit., p. 570.

Guthrie, H.A. "Introductory Nutrition," pp. 243, 245, Mosby, 1971.

Snell, E.E. in "The Vitamins" Vol. III, Op.Cit., p. 387.

Watson, C. Op.Cit.

318. Bourne, G.H. in "Biochemistry and Physiology of Nutrition," Vol. II, p. 104, ed. by Bourne, G.H. and Kidder, G.W., Academic Press, 1953.

Luttrell, C.N. and Mason, K.E. Ann.N.Y. Acad.Sci., 52:113, 1949.

Lipshutz, M.D. Rev.Neurol., 65:221, 1936.

Mason, K.E. in "The Vitamins," Vol. III, Op.Cit., p. 535.

319. Bethell, F.H. in "The Vitamins," Op.Cit., p. 203.

Williams, R.J. "Nutrition Against Disease," p. 161, Bantam, 1973.

Street, H.R., et al. J.Nutr., 21:275, 1941.

Sherman, H. in "The Vitamins," Vol. III, Op.Cit., p. 274.

Follis, R.H. and Wintrobe, M.M. J.Exptl.Med., 81:539, 1945.

Ramalingaswami, V. and Sinclair, H.M. Brit.J.Nutr., 4(2 and 3): xiii, 1950.

320. Hawkins, W.W. and Barsky, J. Science, 108:284, 1948.

Stone, S. Diseases of Nervous System, 11:131, 1950.

321. Cotlove, E. and Hogben, C.A.M. "Mineral Metabolism," Vol. II, Part B, p. 153, ed. by Comar, C.L. and Bronner, F., Academic Press, 1962.

Harrison, H.E., et al. J.Clin.Invest., 31:300, 1952.

Welt, L.G., et al. J.Applied Physiol., 6:134, 1952.

Cort, J.H. Lancet, i:752, 1954.

Adelstein, S.J. and Vallee, B.L. in "Mineral Metabolism," Vol. II, Op.Cit, p. 379.

Underwood, E.J. "Trace Elements in Human and Animal Nutrition," Academic Press, 1956.

323. Swank, R.L. "A biochemical basis of multiple sclerosis" pp. 3, 44–45, Thomas, 1961.

Cheraskin, E. and Ringsdorf, W.M. "New Hope for Incurable Diseases," p. 32, Arco, 1971.

324. Mitchell, D.A. and Schandl, E.K. Am.J.Clin.Nutr., 26(8):890, 1973.

325. Ibid.

326. Noble, R.L., et al. Can.Med.Assn.J., January, 1957.

Abrahamson, E.M. N.Y.State Med.J., 54:11, 1954; 54:1603, 1954.

327. Ibid.

Organic Consumer Report, 52(26), June 27, 1972.

Swank, R.L. "A Bio.Basis for M.S.," Op.Cit., pp. 38–52.

Cooper, L.F., et al. "Nutrition in Health and Disease," p. 536, Lippincott, 1963.

Evers, J. Cancer Control J. 2(3):5, 1974.

Waerland, E. "The Waerland Therapies," Nords. Forlag., 1955.

328. Organic Consumer Report, 52(26), June 27, 1972.

Stone, P. Diseases Nerv. Syst., 11:1, 1950.

Stephens, M.C., et al. J.Neurochem., 18:2407, 1971.

Guthrie, H.A. Op.Cit., pp. 255–256.

Mitchell, D.A. and Schandl, E.K. Am.J.Clin.Nutr., 26(8):890, 1973.

329. Abrahamson, E.M. N.Y. State J.Med., 54:11, 1954.

330. Swank, R.L. Arch.Neurol., 23:466, 1970.

Swank, R.L. and Grimsgaard, A. "Low-fat Diet: Reasons, Rules and Recipes," U.Oregon, 1959.

331. Bernsohn, J., et al. Science News, September 30, 1967.

Cooper, L.F., et al. "Nutrition in Health and Disease," p. 536, Lippincott, 1963.

332. Clark, M. Prevention, November, 1972.

Evers, J. Op.Cit.

334. Swank, R.L. "A Biochemical Basis of Multiple Sclerosis," Op.Cit., p. 32.

Cheraskin, E. and Ringsdorf, W.M. Op.Cit., p. 48.

336. Louisot, P., et al. Clin.Chim.Acta, 48(4):373, 1973.

McQuerrie, I. Encyl.Brit., 5:509, 1969.

337. Lapey, A., et al. J.Pediatr., 84:8328, 1974.

Oppenhimer, E.H. and Esterby, J.R. Arch.Path., 96:149, 1973.

338. Lapey, A., et al. Op.Cit.

McQurrie, I. Op.Cit.

Fish, D. Austin American Statesman, 1974.

References: Chapter IV

340. Leaf, A. Ntl.Geog., 143:93, 1973.

341. Ibid.

Benet, S. N.Y.Times, Dec. 26, 1971.

Armstrong, T. Soil and Health J., Oct.–Nov., 1965.

342. Loma Linda U. School of Health. "Summary of Results of Adventist Mortality Study—1958–65," 1974.

Burn, H. "Our Most Interesting Diseases," pp. 114–115, Scribner's Sons, 1964.

Wall Street J. Apr. 12, 1974.

343. Leaf, A. Op.Cit.

Benet, S. Op.Cit.

Armstrong, T. Op.Cit.

344. Ross, M.H. J.Nutr., 97 (4 Suppl. 1 pt. 2):563, 1969.

345. Ross, M.H. Am.J.Clin.Nutr., 25:834, 1972.

346. Durand, A. Arch.Pathol., 85(3):318, 1968.

McKay, C.M., et al. Arch.Biochem., 2:469, 1943.

French, C.E., et al. J.Nutr., 51:329, 1953.

Silberberg, M. and Silberberg, R. Can J. Biochem.Physiol., 33: 67, 1955.

349. Cartis, H.J. "Biological Mechanisms of Aging," Charles C. Thomas, 1966.

350. Bodansky, O. "Biochemistry of Disease," 2nd ed. p. 784, McMillan, 1952.
Mitchell, H.S., et al. "Cooper's Nutrition in Health and Disease," 15th ed., Lippincott, 1968.

351. Cartis, H.J. "Biological Mechanisms of Aging," Charles C. Thomas, 1966.
Odland, L.M., et al. Am.J.Clin.Nutr., 25:905, 1972.
Albanese, A.A., et al. Nutrition Reports International, 8(2):119, 1973.
Ellis, F.R., et al. Am.J.Clin.Nutr., 25:555, 1972.
Wachman, A. and Bernstein, D.S. Lancet, 1:958, 1968.

352. Newton-John, H.F. and Morgan, D.B. Lancet, 1:232, 1968.
Ellis, F. et al., Am.J.Clin.Nutr., 27:769, 1974.
Benet, S. Op.Cit.

353. Walker, A.K.P., et al. Postgrad.Med.J., 47(548):320, 1971.
Zeegeluar, F.J., et al. Am.J.Clin.Nutr., 20:43, 1967.

355. Wachman, A. and Bernstein, D.S. Op.Cit.
Anand, C.R. and Linkswiler, H.M. J.Nutr., 104:695, 1974.

356. Krook, T., et al. Cornell Vet., 62(3):371, 1972.

357. Shah, B.G., et al. J.Nutr., 92(1):30, 1967.
Draper, H.H., et al. J.Nutr., 102:1133, 1972.
Krishnarao, G.V.G. and Draper, H.H., J.Nutr., 102:1143, 1972.

358. Albanese, A.A., et al. Op.Cit.
Leichsenring, J.M., et al. J.Nutr., 45:407, 1951.
Harrand, R.B. and Hartles, R.L. Brit.J.Nutr., 24(4):929, 1970.

361. Johnson, N.E., et al. J.Nutr., 100(12)1425, 1970.
Walker, R.M. and Linkswiler, H.M. J.Nutr., 102:1297, 1972.

362. Anand, C.R. and Linkswiler, H.M. J.Nutr., 104:695, 1974.

364. Ibid.

365. Irwin, I. and Kienholz, E. J.Nutr., 103:1019, 1973.

366. Begum, A. and Pererira, S. Br. J.Nutr., 23(4):905, 1969.
Hulley, S.B., et al. J.Clin.Invest., 50(12):2506, 1971.
Koshi, F. U.S. Army Med.Nutr.Lab.Rep. no. 211, pp. 1–19, 1957.
Shore, J.D. and Consolazio, C.F. Ibid, no. 241, pp. 1–13, 1959.
Fioria, F., et al. Aerosp.Med., 39:714, 1968.
Eichler, J. Z.Rheumaforsch., 31:367, 1972.

367. Cotzias, G.C. Fed.Proc., 19:655, 1960.

368. Ibid.
Peterson, W.H., et al. "Elements of Food Biochemistry," pp. 267–271, Prentice-Hall, 1946.

369. Benet, S. Op.Cit.
Walker, A.K.P. Op.Cit.
Zeeguluar, F.J., et al. Op.Cit.

372. Francis, M.D. and Brener, W.W. J.Dent.Res., 48(6 part 2):1185, 1969.
Fomon, S.J., et al. Am.J.Clin.Nutr., 23(10):1299, 1971.
Dreizen, S., et al. Invest.Urol., 4(5):445, 1967.
Wohl, M.G. and Goodhart, R.S. "Mod.Nutr. in Health and Disease," 4th ed., Lea and Febiger, 1968.
Goulding, A. and Malthus, R.S. J.Nutr., 97(3):353, 1969.
Jacob, Mary and Forbes, R.M. J.Nutr., 99(1):51, 1969.
Smith, B.S.W. and Nisbet, D.I. J.Comp.Pathol., 82:37, 1972.
McGraw-Hill Encyclopedia of Sci. and Tech., 1960.
Forbes, R.M. J.Nutr., 101(1):35, 1971.

373. Smith, B.S.W. and Nisbet, D.I. J.Comp.Pathol., 82(1):37, 1972.

374. Gershoff, S.N. and Prien, E.L. Am.J.Clin.Nutr., 20(5):393, 1967.
Williams, R.J. "Nutrition Against Disease," p. 82, Bantam Books, 1973.
Britton, W.M. and Stockstad, E.L.R. J.Nutr., 100(12):1501, 1970.

375. Seelig, M.S., Am.J.Clin.Nutr., 14:342, 1964.
Alcock, N., et al. Clin.Sci., 22:185, 1962.
Knapp, C.L. J.Clin.Invest., 26:182, 1947.
Guthrie, H.A., "Introductory Nutrition," pp. 109, 110, 118, 206, Mosby, 1971.

376. Ibid, p. 135.

377. Miyake, H. and Johnston, C.G. Digestion, 1:219, 1968.
Kameda, H. Gastroenterology, 46:109, 1964.

379. Encyl.Brit., 2:515, 1968.

381. Williams, R.J. Op.Cit., p. 134.
Roberts, J. and Burch, T.A. U.S.Pub.Health Ser.Pub.No. 1000, Series 11, No. 5, 1966.
Benet, S., Op.Cit.

382. Blaw, S.P. and Schultz, D. "Arthritis," Doubleday, 1974.

383. Turner, D. "Handbook of Diet Therapy," U.Chicago, 1959.

384. Kim, J.C. and Cohen, A.S. Proc.Soc.Exptl.Bio.Med., 123:77, 1966.
Chung, A.C., et al. Arthritis and Rheum., 5:176, 1962.

385. Silberberg, M. and Silberberg, R. Arch.Path., 50:828, 1950; 70:385, 1960.
Sokloff, L. "The Biology of Degenerative Joint Disease," U. Chicago, 1969.
Rubens-Duval, A., et al. Path.Biol., 5:1649, 1957.
Kuzell, W.C. Ann.Rev.Med., 2:367, 1951.

386. Greenberg, L.D. and Rinehart, J.F. Proc.Soc.Exp.Biol.Med., 76:580, 1951.

Ellis, J.M. "The Doctor Who Looked at Hands," ARC Books, 1966.

Barton-Wright, E.G. and Elliot, N.A. Lancet, p. 862, Oct. 26, 1963.

Stephens, C.S., et al. Ann.Inter.Med., 27:420, 1967.

391. Spiera, H., et al. Brit.J.Dermatol., 85(3):277, 1971.

Petrozyi, J.W. and Rosenbloom, J.J.A.M.A., 205(6):345, 1968.

394. Jedziniak, J.A., et al. Invest.Ophth., 11(11):905, 1972.

Berlyne, G.M., et al. Lancet, 1(7749):509, 1972.

Pau, H. Albrecht Von Graefes Arch.Klin.Exp.Ophth., 186:165, 1973.

Bunce, G.E., et al. Proc.Soc.Exp.Biol.Med., 140(3):1103, 1972.

395. Ferguson, T.M. et al. Proc.Soc.Exp.Biol.Med., 86:868, 1954.

Ibid. AMA.Arch.Ophthal., 55:346, 1956.

Gardiner, P.A. Dev.Med.Child Neurol., 14:661, 1972.

396. York, A.T., et al. Ophthalmic Res., 2(5):273, 1971.

Fournier, D.J. and Patterson, J.W. Proc.Soc.Exp.Bio.Med., 137(3):826, 1971.

Srivastava, S.K. and Beutler, E. Biochem.Med., 6(4):372, 1972.

Van Heyningen, R. Exp.Eye Res., 11(3):415, 1971.

397. Ibid.

Reddy, V.N. Exp. Eye Res., 11(3):310, 1971.

Dawidowicz, A. Waid Lek., 24(6):545, 1971.

Marquardt, R. and Krischbaum, H. Klin.Monatsbl.Augenheilkd. 159:769, 1971.

Lakowski, R., et al. Ophthalmic Res., 4(3):145, 1972/1973.

398. Frenkel, G. Diabetologia, 8(5):313, 1972.

Mueller, F.O. Z.Gesamte.Hyg.Grenzgeb., 19:861, 1971.

Dudenko, N.V. Vopr.Okhr.Mater.Det., 14(9):83, 1969.

Katsumata, R. Nagoya J.Med.Sci., 32:261, 1970.

Singh, I. Lancet 268:422, 1955.

Larsson, S. Acta Physiol.Scand. Suppl. 294, pp. 7–82, 1967.

399. Agzamova, Kh.S. Zdravookhr.Turkm., 16(1):30, 1972.

Swinson, R.P. Br.J.Physiol.Opt., 27(1):43, 1972.

Sopek, M. and Slizewski, M. Neurdl.Neurochir.Pol., 22:269, 1972.

Miszke, A. Folia Med.Cracov., 14(1):29, 1972.

Ivanova-Chemeshanska, L. Gig.Sanit., 36(11):95, 1971.

400. Malika, K., et al. Otolaryngol.Pol., 26:309, 1972.

Schmitz-Valckenberg, P. Albrecht Von Graefes Arch.Klin.Exp. Ophth., 186(4):339, 1973.

DeLorenzo, A.J. and Darin, A.J. Ed., "Vascular Disorders and

Hearing Defects," U.Park Press., 1973.

Karvonen, M.J. Proc.Nutr.Soc., 31:355, 1972.

Eivazov, A.A. Vestn.Otorinol., 34(2):17, 1972.

Senzukov, M.V. Vestn.Otorinol., 34(2):20, 1972.

402. Berman, P.M. and Kussmer, I.B. Am.J.Dig.Dis., 17(8): 741, 1972.

403. Robinson, C.H. "Normal and Therapeutic Nutrition," 13th Ed., p. 386, MacMillan, 1967.

404. Cowgill, G.R. and Ander, W.E. J.A.M.A., 98:1866, 1932.

Hardinge, M.G., et al. Am.J.Clin.Nutr., 6:523, 1958.

405. Berman, P.M. and Kirsner, J.B. Am.J.Dig.Dis., 17(8):741, 1972.

406. Berry, W.H. Colliers Encyl.

411. Barberas, R.F. Gastro., 65(6):1168, 1973.

414. Anisimov, V.E. Bio.Abs. 126457, 52(22):12616, 1971.

Samson, E.I. Ibid 1244, 55(1):143, 1973.

Snegireva, F.V., et al. Prikl.Biokhim., Mikrobiol., 9(2):179, 1973.

415. Jolliffe, N., et al. "Chemical Nutrition," Harper, 1950.

416. St.John, D.J.B. Gastro., 65:634, 1973.

McDonald, W.C. Ibid, 65:381, 1973.

Pare, W.P. and Hauser, V.P. Bull Psychonomic Soc., 2(4):213, 1973.

References: Chapter V

428. Hegsted, D.M. in "Nutrition," Vol. I, ed. by Beaton, G.H. and McHenry, E.W., pp. 125–126, Academic Press, 1964.

441. Kofranzi, E., et al. Hoppe-Seylers Z. Physol.Chem., 351(12): 1485, 1970.

442. Ibid.

Kies, C. and Fox, H. Cereal Chem., 47(5):615, 1970.

Ibid. J.Fd.Sci., 38(7):1211, 1973.

Clark, H., et al. Am.J.Clin.Nutr., 26(7):702, 1973.

Clark, H., et al. J.Nutr., 102:1647, 1972.

Edwards, C.H., et al. Am.J.Clin.Nutr., 24(2):181, 1971.

Leverton, R.M., et al. J.Nutr., 58(1):59, 1956.

Lee, C.-J., et al. Am.J.Clin.Nutr., 24(3):318, 1971.

Inoue, G., et al. J.Nutr., 103(12):1673, 1973.

Taylor, Y., et al. Br.J.Nutr., 32(2):407, 1974.

443. Calloway, D.H. and Spector, H. Am.J.Clin.Nutr., 2(6):405, 1954.

Inoue, G., Op.Cit.

Naismith, D.J. and Holdsworth, M.D. Proc.Nutr. Soc., 29(2): 55A, 1970.

444. Scrimshaw, N.S., et al. Am.J.Clin.Nutr., 26(9):965, 1973.

Inoue, G., et al. Op.Cit.

Kofranzi, E., et al. Op.Cit.

446. U.S. Dept. of Agriculture Household Food Consumption Survey Report #6, March, 1957.

448. Chittenden, R.H. "Physiol.Econ. in Nutr.," Stokes, 1904.

Pettenkofer, M. and Voit, C. Z.Biol., 2, 1866.

Chaney, M.S. and Ross, M.L. "Nutrition," 7th Ed., pp. 104–105, Houghton Mifflin, 1966.

Christensen, E.H. "Das Essen und trinken des Sportlers. Sportmedizinsche Schuftenreihe," Bern:Wanderer, 1958.

Astand, P.O. Fed. Proc., 26(6):1772, 1957.

Hedman, R. Acta Physiol.Scand., 40:305, 1957.

Karlsson, J. and Saltin, B. J.Appl.Physiol., 3:203, 1971.

Ahrens, R.A. and Wilson, J.E. J.Nutr., 90(1):63, 1966.

Bjorntorp, P. et al. Hormone Metab.Res., 4(3):182, 1972.

Henhede, M. "Protein and Nutrition," Ewart, Seymour, 1913.

449. Ashworth, Ann and Harrower, A.D.B. Brit. J.Nutr., 21(4):833, 1967.

450. Bergstrom, J., et al. Acta Physiol. Scand., 71:140, 1967.

Karlsson, J. and Saltin, B. Op.Cit.

Kvartovkina, L.K. and Minkh, A.A. Gig.Sanit., 33(3):75, 1968.

Fuge, K.W., et al. Am.J.Physiol., 215(3):660, 1968.

Barboriak, J.J. and Wilson, A.S. J.Nutr., 102:1543, 1972.

Ahrens, R.A. and Wilson, J.E. Op.Cit.

Canolazio, C.F. et al. Am.J.Clin.Nutr., 25:85, 1972.

451. Hegsted, D.M. Op.Cit., p. 170.

Cuthbertson, D.P. Quat.J.Med. (N.S.), 1:233, 1932.

Ibid, Brit.J.Surg., 23:505, 1936.

Calloway, D.H., et al. Surgery, 37:935, 1955.

452. Hansen, J.E., et al. J.Appl.Philsiol., 33:441, 1972.

Schnakenberg, D.D. Proc.Soc.Exp.Bio.Med., 134(4):905, 1970.

455. Mikelsen, Olaf, et al. J.Nutr., 57:541, 1955.

U.S. Dept. of Agr. "Composition of Foods," Handbook #8, pp. 13, 18, Revised 1963.

456. Stein, J.M., et al. Metab.Clin.Exp., 20:903, 1971.

Sack, M.J. Proc.Nutr.Soc., 31:15A, 1972.

Miller, D.S. and Parsonage, S.R. Proc.Nutr.Soc., 31:31A, 1972.

457. Kempner, W. N.Car.Med.J., 5:125, 1944.
Watkins, D.M., et al. Am.J.Med., 9:428, 1950.
Williamson, C.R. N.E.J.Med., 243, 1977, 1950.
Chapman, C.B. N.E.J.Med., 243:899, 1950.
Currens, J.H., et al. N.E.J.Med., 245:354, 1951.
Dole, V.P., et al. J.Clin.Invest., 29:1187, 1950.
Page, I.H. and Corcoran, A.C. J.Clin.Nutr., 1:7, 1952.
Møller, E. Acta Med.Scand., 74:341, 1931.
Dole, V.P., et al. Am.J.Clin.Nutr., 2(6):381, 1954.
460. Benke, P.J. Biochem.Med., 6(6):526, 1972.
Margen, S., et al. Am.J.Clin.Nutr., 27(6):584, 1974.
461. Kasper, H. Uschau.Wiss.Tech., 67(10):328, 1967.
Suzuki, S., et al. Ann.Rep.Nat.Inst.Nutr., pp. 1–9, 1967.
462. Ross, M.H. J.Nutr., 97(4 Suppl. 1 Part 2):563, 1969.
463. Ross, M.H. Am.J.Clin.Nutr., 25:834, 1972.
Ibid. Fed.Proc., 18:1190, 1959.
464. Watanbe, T. et al. Acta Med.Nagasaki, 13:44, 1968.
Acsaki, Gy., and Memeskeri, J. "History of Human Life Span and Mortality," Akademicai Kcado, Budapest, 1970.
Jose, D.G. and Good, R.A. Cancer Res., 33:807, 1973.
Armstrong, T. Soil and Health J. (New Zealand), Oct.–Nov., 1965.
465. Anderson, D.E., et al. J.Nat.Cancer Inst., 45:697, 1970.
466. Bagchi, K., et al. Am.J.Clin.Nutr., 13(4):232, 1963.
Hardinge, M.C. and Stare, F.J. J.Clin.Nutr., 2:73, 1954.
West, R.O. and Hayes, O.B. Am.J.Clin.Nutr., 23:249, 1970.
Krause, M.V. "Food, Nutrition and Diet Therapy," 3rd Ed., 1961.
Blacket, R.B. Postgrad.Med.J., 46(534):221, 1970.
Mann, G.V., et al. J.Atherosclerosis Res., 4:289, 1964.
467. Sukhatme, P.V. Brit.J.Nutr., 24(2):477, 1970.
Saheki, T. Shik.Acta Med., 28:292, 1972.
Nuzum, C.T., et al. Science (Washington), 172(3987):1042, 1971.
Bolourchi, S., et al. Am.J.Clin.Nutr., 21(8):827, 1968.
Edwards, C.H., et al. Am.J.Clin.Nutr., 24(2):181, 1971.
468. Dimitriu, C.G., et al. Med.Interna, 23(9):1055, 1971.
Giordano, C.R., et al. Proc.Int.Cong.Nephrol., 3:214, 1966.
Giovannetti, S., Proc.Int.Cong.Nephrol., 3:230, 1966.
Bergeron, Michel-G. Laval Med., 41(3):340, 1970.
470. Nagy, M. J.A.M.A., Vol. 226, Nov. 19, 1973.
deWardener, H.C. "The Kidney," p. 230, Little Brown and Co., 1958.
Bergman, F. et al. Acta Chir.Scand., 132(6):715, 1966.
Ibid. Bio.Abs. 21392,52:2237, 1971.

471. Turner, D. "Handbook of Diet Therapy" 4th Ed., U.Chicago Press, 1965.
472. Spiera, H., et al. Brit.J.Dermatol., 85(3):277, 1971.
     Shamov, I.A. Vopr.Pitan., 29(5):40, 1970.
     Rich, L.F., et al. Exp.Eye Res., 17(1):87, 1973.
     Mitchell, H.S. and Cook, G.M. Proc.Soc.Exptl.Biol.Med., 36:806, 1937.
     Hall, W.K., et al. J.Nutr., 36:277, 1948.
473. Johnson, N.E., et al. J.Nutr., 100(12):1425, 1970.
     Walker, R. and Linkswiler, H., J.Nutr., 102:1297, 1972.
476. Guthrie, H.A. "Introductory Nutrition," 2nd Ed., p. 48, Mosby, 1971.
477. Silberberg, M., et al. Can.J.Biochem.Physiol., 33:167, 1955.
     French, C.E., et al. Am.J.Physio., 123:526, 1938.
     Watson, A.F., et al. Brit.J.Exptl.Pathol., 11:311, 1930.
     Lavik, P.S., et al. Cancer Res., 3:748, 1943.
     Rasch, et al. Cancer Res., 5:431, 1945.
     Silverstone, H., et al. Cancer Res., 9:354, 1949.
     Kirby, A.H.M. Cancer Res., 5:129, 1945.
     Newsweek. Feb. 18, 1974.
     Am.Cancer Soc.News, 25:13, 1971.
     Wynder, W.L. N.Y.Post, Jan. 24, 1974.
     Singh, I. Lancet, 268:422, 1955.
     Rains, A.J.H.Encyl.Am., 12:253, 1971.
     "Cooper's Nutrition in Health and Disease," 15th Ed., Lippincott, 1968.
     Swank, R.L. Arch. Neurol., 23:466, 1970.
478. Miller, D.S. and Parsonage, S.R. Proc.Soc.Nutr., 31:31A, 1972.
     Larsson, S. Acta Physiol.Scand., Suppl. 294, pp. 7–82, 1967.
     J.Nutr., 100(9):104, 1970.
     Velichko, A.A. Vopr.Pitan., 25:76, 1966.
     Lemonnier, D., et al. Ann. Nutr.Aliment., 22:107, 1968.
     DiCostanzo, G. Arch.Sci.Physiol., 24:337, 1970.
     Schemmel, R., et al. J.Nutr., 102:1187, 1972.
     Leaf, A. Natl.Geog., Jan., 1973.
     Kinderlehrer, J. Prevention, 26(5):77, 1974.
480. Huzar, G. Vitalst.Zivilisation Skr., 10(50):207, 1965.
482. Kofranzi, E., et al. Op.Cit.
     Graham, G.G., et al. Am.J.Clin.Nutr., 25(9):875, 1973.
     Whohl, M.S. and Goodhart, R.S. "Modern Nutrition in Health and Disease," chapter 6, 4th Ed., Lea and Febiger, 1968.
     Doraisvamy, T.R., et al. Brit.J.Nutr., 23(4):737, 1963.

484. Elias, L.G., et al. Arch.Latinoamer.Nutr. 19(2):109, 1969.
     Alvi, A.S., et al. Pakistan J.Med.Res., 7(3):207, 1967.
     Pereira, S., et al. J.Food Sci.Tech., 5(3):133, 1968.
     DeOliveira, J.E.D. Arch.Latinoamer.Nutr., 17(3):197, 1967.
485. Burkholder, R.R. Science, June 18, 1943.
     Tabekhia, M.M., et al. Nutr.Abs. and Rev. 3607, 43(6):466, 1973.
     Shorey, R.L. Personal Communication, June 7, 1974.
486. Atkinson, J. and Carpenter, K.J. Proc.Nutr., Soc. 29:56A, 1970.
     Pronczuk, A., et al. Nutr.Metab., 15(3):171, 1973.
487. Juliano, B.O., et al. Cereal Chem. Today, 13(8):299, 1968.
     Srinivasan, K.S., et al. J.Food Sci.Techol., 7(2):95, 1970.
     Yannai, S. and Zimmermann, G. Cereal Chem., 48(1):40, 1971.
     Bourges, H., et al. Nutr.Rep.Int., 4(1):31, 1971.
     Burlacu, G., et al. Stud.Ceret.Biol.Ser.Zool., 21(1):77, 1969.
     Cravioto, B., et al. Ciencia, 24(12):83, 1965.
     Srinivasan, P.C., et al. J.Nutr.Diet., 6(3):192, 1969.
     J.Agr.Food Chem., 17(4):791, 1969.
     Ahsan, R., et al. Pak.J.Biochem., 1:16, 1968.
     Cerney, K., et al. Brit.J.Nutr., 26(2):293, 1971.
488. Scrimshaw, N.S., et al. Am.J.Clin.Nutr., 26:965, 1973.
     Ghai, O.P. and Chaudhuri, S.N. Indian J.Med.Res., 59(5):756, 1971.
     Efremov, V.V., et al. Gig.Sanit., 35(6):88, 1970.
     Trigg, T.E. and Topps, J.H. Proc.Soc.Nutr., 31:45A, 1972.
     Abernathy, R.P., et al. Am.J.Clin.Nutr., 25(10):980, 1972.
     Periera, S.M., et al. Brit.J.Nutr., 30(2):241, 1973.
492. Chaney, M.S. and Ross, M.L. "Nutrition," 7th Ed., pp. 379, 381, Houghton-Mifflin, 1966.
     Williams, R.J. "Nutrition in a Nutshell," p. 86, Dolphin Books, 1962.
     Davis, A. "Let's Have Healthy Children," p. 139, Signet Books, 1972.
493. McCance, R.A. and Widdowson, E.M. "The Composition of Foods," pp. 5, 33, Her Maj.Stat.Office, 1960.
494. Chaney, M.S. and Ross, M.L. Op.Cit., p. 393.
495. Matoth, Y., et al. Am.J.Clin.Nutr., 21(3):226, 1968.
     Elias, L.G., et al. Arch.Latinoamer.Nutr., 19:109, 1969.
     Beghin, I., et al. Am.J.Clin.Nutr., 26:246, 1973.

496. Sterns, G. Physiol.Rev., 19:415, 1939.
Holt, L.E., Jr., et al. "Protein and Amino Acid Requirements in Early Life," N.Y. Univ.Press., 1960.
Guthrie, H.A., Op.Cit. p. 349.
Hegsted, D.M. in "Nutrition," Vol. I, ed. by Beaton, G.H. and McHenry, E.W., p. 142, Academic Press, 1964.
Alvi, A.S., et al. Pakistan J.Med.Res., 7(3):207, 1967.
Oelshegel, F.J. Jr., et al. J.Agr.Food Chem., 17(4):791, 1969.
Doraiswamy, T.R., et al. Br.J.Nutr., 23(4):737, 1969.
Burlacu, G., et al. Stud.Ceret, Biol.Ser.Zool., 21(1):77, 1969.

References: Chapter VI

505. Guthrie, H.A. "Introductory Nutrition," 2nd Ed., p. 117, Mosby, 1971.
Watt, B.K. and Merrill, A.F. "Composition of Foods," U.S.D.A. Agriculture Handbook No. 8, p. 162, Revised, 1963.
506. Jelliffe, D.B. Pl.Fds.Hum.Nutr., 2:145, 1972.
Ibid. "Child Nutrition in Developing Countries," USDHEW, 1968.
Ibid. World Health Org. (U.N.) Monograph No. 23, Geneva, 1968.
508. Schwegirt, B.S., et al. J.Nutr., 29:405, 1945.
McCay, C.M. and Easton, E.M. J.Nutr., 34:351, 1947.
513. Guthrie, H.A. Op.Cit, pp. 205–206.
Taylor, A.N. and Wasserman, R.H. Fed.Proc., 28(6):1834, 1969.
514. U.S.D.A. Handbook No. 8, p. 133.
Guthrie, H.A. Op.Cit., pp. 210–211.
Patzelt-Wenczler, R. Nutr. Abs.Rev., 43(2):112, 1973.
Berénshtéîn, G.F. Nutr.Abs.Rev. 4466,43(7):554, 1973.
Cheeke, P.R. and Shull, L.R.A. Nutr.Rep.Intr., 6(2):93, 1972.
Williams, R.J. "Nutrition Against Disease," pp. 254–255, Bantam Books, 1973.
Chen, L.H., et al. J.Nutr., 102(6):729, 1972.
Stuffel, P. Canad.Med.Assoc.J., 74:715, 1956.
Ehrlich, H.P., et al. Nutr.Abs.Rev. 962, 43(2):111, 1973.
Evarts, R.P. and Oksanen, A. Brit.J.Nutr., 29(2):293, 1973.
Villers, A. et al. Nutr.Abs.Rev., 155, 44(1):16, 1974.
Noguchi, T. et al. Agr.Bio.Chem., 36(10):1667, 1972.
Guthrie, H.A. Op.Cit., p. 213.
Lipshutz, M.D. Rev.Neurol., 65:221, 1936.

Luttrell, C.N. and Mason, K.E. Ann.N.Y.Acad.Sci., 52:113, 1949.

Bourne, G.H. in "Biochemistry and Physiology of Nutrition," Vol. II, p. 104, ed. by Bourne, G.H. and Kidder, G.W. Academic Press, 1953.

515. Hazell, K. and Baloch, K.H. Gerontol.Clin., 12:10, 1970.
Lovric, V.A., et al. Aust.N.Z.J.Med., 1(1):35, 1971.

516. Follis, R.H. "The Pathology of Nutritional Diseases," Blackwell, 1948.
Brozek, J. Am.J.Clin.Nutr., 5:109, 1957.
Guthrie, H.A. Op.Cit., pp. 243, 245, Mosby, 1971.

517. Shaw, J.H. and Phillips, P.H. J.Nutr., 22:345, 1941.
Engel, R.W. and Phillips, P.H. Proc.Soc.Exptl.Biol.Med., 46: 597, 1939.

518. Chaney, M.S. and Ross, M.L. "Nutrition" 7th Ed., pp. 281–284, 292–293, Houghton Mifflin, 1966.
Hundley, J.M. in "The Vitamins," Vol. II, ed by Sebrell, W.H. and Harris, R.S., p. 570, Academic Press, 1954.

520. Cohenour, S.H. and Calloway, D.H. Am.J.Clin.Nutr., 25:512, 1972.

521. Bridgers, W.F. Nutr.Rev., 25:65, 1967.
Sebrell, H.S., Jr. and Harris, R.S. in "The Vitamins," Vol. 1, Op.Cit., p. 525.

523. Guthrie, H.A. Op.Cit., pp. 255–256.
Stephens, M.C., et al. J.Neurochem., 18(12):2407, 1971.
Chow, B.F. in "Nutrition," Vol. II, ed. by Beaton, G.H. and McHenry, E.W., pp. 212, 214, Academic Press, 1964.
Sprince, H., Nutr.Rep.Int., 1(4):243, 1970.
Review. Nutr.Rev., 21:143, 1963.
Hinse, C.M. and Lupien, R.J. Can.J.Biochem., 49(8):933, 1971.

524. Chaney, M.S. and Ross, M.L. Op.Cit., p. 302.
Axelrod, A.E. Am.J.Clin.Nutr., 24:261, 1971.
Leuchtenberger, R. "Approaches to Tumor Chemotherapy," p. 163, Am.Assoc. for the Advancement of Science, 1947.
Guthrie, H.A. Op.Cit., p. 207.
Alperin, J.B., et al. Arch.Inter.Med., 117:681, 1966.
Lindenbaum, J. and Klipstein, F.A. J.Clin.Path. 17:666, 1964.

527. Krebs, E.T. Cancer News J., May/Aug., 1970.
Kinderlehrer, J. Prevention, 26(5):77, 1974.

528. Watson, M. Personal Communication, August, 1974.
Kemp, G.L. J.Am.Osteo.Assoc., 58:714, 1959.
Pettigrew, A.L. Ibid, 59:968, 1960.
Schmulych, V.K. and Loboda, M.V. Ped.Akush.Hinekol., 33(6):22, 1971.

Beard, Howard. "A New Approach to the Conquest of Cancer, Rheumatic and Heart Diseases, Pageant Press, 1958.

Kutateladge, E.A. and Dzhabua, M.I. Soobhch.Akad.Nauk. Gruz. S.S.R., 57(3):737, 1970.

Vashchuck, A.S., et al. Bio.Abs. 32904, 53(6):3270, 1972.

Udalov, Yu.F. and Sokolova, M.M. Bio.Abs. 10004, 45:804, 1964.

Santi, P., Bio.Abs. 67437, 36:6293, 1961.

529.   Anisimov, V.E. Bio.Abs. 126457, 52(22):12616, 1971.

Samson, E.I. Bio.Abs. 1244,55(1):143, 1973.

530.   Watson, M. Op.Cit.

Drasar, B.S. and Hill, M.J. Am.J.Clin.Nutr., 25:1394, 1973.

Bishop, J.E. Wall St.J., Oct. 23, 1973.

Balmer, J. and Zilversmit, D.B. J.Nutr., 104(10):1319, 1974.

540.   Hanssen, M. "About the Salt of Life," pp. 19–20, 27, Thorsons, 1968.

Liechti-v. Brasch, D., et al. "Bircher-Benner Salt Free Nutrition Plan," p. 16, Nash, 1972.

Bieler, H.G. "Food is Your Best Medicine," pp. 219–220, Vintage, 1965.

541.   Consolazio, C.F., et al. J.Nutr., 79:407, 1963.

Guthrie, H.A. Op.Cit., p. 128.

543.   Ibid., p. 154.

Chaney, M.S. and Ross, M.L. Op.Cit., pp. 165, 174.

544.   Ibid., p. 177.

Smith, B.S.W. and Nesbit, D.L. Bio.Abs. 98791, 49(9):8876, 1968.

Dunn, M. and Walser, M. Metab. Clin.Exp., 15(10):884, 1966.

548.   Scott, D.E. and Pritchard, J.A. J.A.M.A., 199(12):897, 1967.

Jeans, P.C., et al. J.Am.Diet.Assn., 28:27, 1952.

549.   Chaney, M.S. and Ross, M.L., Op.Cit., pp. 150, 179, 140–1.

Muller, H.B. Virchows. Arch.Abt.A.Pathol.Anat., 350(4):353, 1970.

Carlton, W.W. and Kelly, W.A. J.Nutr., 97(1):42, 1969.

Smolyar, V.I., Bio.Abs. 70779, 51:6930, 1970.

550.   Seelig, M.S., Am.J.Clin.Nutr., 26:657, 1973.

Schroeder, H.A., et al. J.Chron.Dis., 23(7):481, 1970.

Guthrie, H.A. Op.Cit., p. 165.

551.   Orent, E.R., et al. J.Biol.Chem., 92:651, 1931.

Keith, T.B., et al. J.Animal Sci., 1:120, 1942.

Johnson, S.R. Ibid, 2:14, 1943.

Bentley, O.G. and Phillips, P.H. J.Dairy Sci., 34:396, 1951.

Barnes, L.L. Proc.Soc.Exptl.Biol.Med., 46:562, 1941.

Cotzias, G.C. Fed.Proc., 19:655, 1960.

References: Chapter VII

567. Makhamadyhanov, I. Bio.Abs. 52544, 57(10):5610, 1974.
570. Texas Department of Agriculture and U.S.D.A. "1973 Texas Field Crop Statistics," Bulletin 106, March, 1974.
   Ibid. "1972 Texas Vegetable Statistic" Bulletin 110, May, 1974.
572. Anderson, James R. "A Geography of Agriculture," pp. 54, 58, Brown, 1970.
   Ibid, p. 54.
573. Ibid., pp. 30, 43.
574. Ibid.
575. Ibid., p. 44.
   Brown, L.R. "Man, Land and Food: Looking Ahead to World Food Needs," p. 27, USDA, 1963.
   Chaney, M.S. and Ross, M.A. "Nutrition," 7th Ed., Houghton Mifflin, 1966.
   Kinderlehrer, J. Prevention, 26(5):77, 1974.
576. Dallas Morning News, p. 1 E., Saturday, July 27, 1974.
580. Anderson, James R. Op.Cit., p. 30.
583. Gajalakshmi, R. and Ramaknshnan, C.V. Pl.Fds.Hom.Nutr., 1: 79, 1969.
596. Mayer, L.U. and Hargrove, S.H. CAED Report #38, 1972.
599. Goldsmith, E., et al. The Ecologist, 2(1):1, 1972.
   Levine, R.J. Wall St.J., Dec. 26, 1973.

References: Appendix IV.

Partial List of Sources Used in Computing Nutrient Content of Foods.

McCance, R.A. and Widdowson, E.M. "The Composition of Foods," Her Majesty's Stationary Office, 1960, with Amendments, 1967.
Peterson, W.H., et al. "Elements of Food Biochemistry," Prentice-Hall, 1946.
Watt, B.K. and Merrill, A.L. "Composition of Foods," Agr.Handbook No. 8, U.S. Dept. Agr., Revised December, 1963.
Hardinge, M.G. and Crooks, H. J.Am.Diet Assoc., 38:240, 1961.
Guthrie, H.A. "Introductory Nutrition," 2nd Ed., Mosby, 1970.
Chaney, M.S. and Ross, M.L. "Nutrition," 7th Ed., Houghton Mifflin, 1966.
Williams, R.J. "Nutrition Against Disease," pp. 351–6, Bantam Books, 1973.
Burkholder, P.R. Science (Wash.), June 18, 1943.

Tabekhia, M.M. and Mohamed, M.S. Alexandria J.Agr.Res., 19(2):285, 1971.

Santini, R., et al. Am.J.Clin.Nutr., 14:205, 1964.

Bunnell, R.H., et al. Ibid, 17(1):1, 1965.

Herting, D.C. and Drury, E.J.E. J.Nutr., 81(4):335, 1963.

Collins, R.A., et al. Ibid, 43(2):313, 1951.

Anisimov, V.E. Kaz.Med.Zh., 2:84, 1970.

Booth, V.H. and Bradford, M.D. Brit. J.Nutr., 17:575, 1963.

Macy, I.G. "The Composition of Milks," Natl.Acad.Sci.-Natl.Res.Council., Pub. 254, Revised, 1953.

Mills, L.D. Ecologist, 3(6):232, 1973.

Chapman, V.J. "Seaweeds," 2nd Ed. pp. 7, 70, 87, 95, 100, Methven, 1970.

Food and Agr.Org. of United Nations and U.S. Dept. Health Education and Welfare. "Food Composition Table for Use in East Asia," Dec., 1972.

Jukes, T.H. and Williams, W.L. in "The Vitamins," Vol. 1, pp. 478–9, Ed. by Sebrell, W.H. and Harris, R.S., Academic Press, 1954.

Kinderlehrer, J. Prevention, 26(5):81, 1974.

Zook, E.G., et al. Cereal Chem., 46(6):720, 1970.

Schroeder, H.A. Am.J.Clin.Nutr., 21(3):230, 1968.

Scott, M.L. J.Nutr., 103:803, 1973.

Chopra, J.G. and Kevany, J. Am.J.Clin.Nutr., 23(2): 231, 1970.

Kamalanathan, G., et al. Indian J.Nutr.Diet., 9(4):202, 1972.

Childelin, V.A., et al. J.Nutr., 26:477, 1943.

Vyayagopalan, P. and Karup, P.A. Athero., 11:257, 1970.

Some Research Findings Showing How Excesses of Fat, Refined Foods, Protein, Salt, etc. Boost Needs for Specific Nutrients.

Misra, H.N. and Fallowfield, J.M., Postgrad Med. J., 47:624, 1971.

Woodard, J.C. Am.J.Pathol., 65(1):269, 1971.

Harper, A.E., et al. J.Agr.Fd.Chem., 5:754, 1957.

Huttunen, J.K. Postgrad Med. J., 47(552):654, 1971.

Huttuned, J.K. Bio.Abs. 55892, 53(10):5500, 1972.

Muskat, E. and Keller, W. Int.Z.Vitaminforsch., 38(5):538, 1968.

Ewen, L. J.Nutr., 93(4):470, 1967.

Muto, S. and Chihoko, M. J.Nutr., 28(3):327, 1972.

Nakamura, T., et al. Tohoku J.Exp.Med., 93(3):227, 1967.

Leuchtenberger, R. "Approaches to Tumor Chemotherapy," p. 163, Am. Assoc. for the Advancement of Science, 1947.

Shojinia, A.M., et al. Nutr.Abs.Rev., 43(6):468, 1973.

Contostavlos, D.L. Lancet, Nov. 24, 1973, p. 1200.

Fox, M.R.S., et al. J.Nutr., 68:371, 1959.

Nath, M.C. and Nath, N. J.Vitamiol. (Osaka), 13(3):239, 1967.

Sivakumar, B., et al. J.Vitamiol. (Osaka), 15(2):151, 1969.

Carre, L., et al. Nutr. Dieta., 11(4):241, 1969.

Alperin, J.B., et al. Blood J. Hematol., 36(5):632, 1970.

Witting, L.A. Am.J.Clin.Nutr., 25(3):257, 1972.

Phillips, P.H. and Engel, R.W. J.Nutr. 16:451, 1938.

Shaw, J.H. and Phillips, P.H. J.Nutr., 22:345, 1941.

Engel, R.W. and Phillips, P.H. Proc.Soc.Exptl.Biol.Med., 40:597, 1939.

Shastri, N.V. and Nath, M.C. Nutr.Abs.Rev. 7209, 43(11):864, 1973.

Bridgers, W.F., Nutr.Rev. 25:65, 1967.

Sebrell, H.S., Jr., and Harris, R.S. in "The Vitamins," Vol. 1, Op.Cit., p. 525.

Gries, Christian L. J.Nutr., 102:1259, 1972.

Sarma, P.S., et al. J.Bio.Chem., 165:55, 1946.

Sastry, G.N.Y. Mysore J. Agr.Sci., 2(1):6, 1968.

Andrieux-Domont, C. and Hang, L.V. Arch.Sci.Physiol., 25(1):47, 1971.

Muller, H.B. Virchows, Arch.Abt.A.Pathol.Anat., 350(4):353, 1970.

Seelig, M.S. Am.J.Clin.Nutr., 26:657, 1973.

Forbes, G.B. in "Mineral Metabolism," Vol. II, Part B. ed by Comar, C.L. and Bronner, F., Academic Press, 1962.

Consolazio, C.F., et al. J.Nutr., 79:407, 1963.

Schroeder, H.A. Am.J.Clin.Nutr., 21(3):230, 1968.

Deshmukh, D.S., et al. Can.J.Physiol.Pharmacol., 48(8):503, 1970.

Some Studies Indicating Persons Taking Normal Diets Are Inclined to Experience Specific Deficiencies.

Shils, M. Am.J.Clin.Nutr., 15(9):133, 1964.

Manalo, R. and Jones, J.E. Am.J.Clin.Nutr., 18:339, 1966.

Osis, D. Am.J.Clin.Nutr., 25:582, 1972.

Scott, D.E. and Pritchard, J.A. J.A.M.A., 199(12):897, 1967.

Basu, R.N., et al. Am.J.Clin.Nutr., 26:591, 1973.

Schroeder, H.A., et al. J.Chron.Dis., 23(7):481, 1970.

Hazell, K. and Baloch, K.H. Gerontol.Clin. 12:10, 1970.

Lovric, V.A., et al. Aust. N.Z.J.Med., 1(1):35, 1971.

Cohenour, S.H. and Calloway, D.H. Am.J.Clin.Nutr., 25:512, 1972.

Bieri, J.G., et al. J.Am.Diet.Assn., 62(2):147, 1973.

Bunnell, R.H., et al. Am.J.Clin.Nutr., 17(1):1, 1965.

Ellis, F.R. and Montegriffo, V.M., Am.J.Clin.Nutr., 23(3):249, 1970.

Kutateladge, E.A. and Dzhabua, M.I. Soobhch.Akad.Nauk.Gruz. S.S.R. 57(3):737, 1970.

Shojinia, A.M., et al. Nutr.Abs.Rev., 43(6):468, 1973.
Gade, S., et al. Nutr.Abs.Rev. 5898, 43(9):704, 1973.
Review: Folacin Activity in U.S. Diet., Nutr.Rev., 22:142, 1964.
Smolyar, V.I. Vopr.Pitan., 28(4):19, 1969.
Sprince, Herbert, Nutr.Rep.Int., 1(4):243, 1970.

Some Important Findings on Needs for Specific Nutrients

Herbert, V. Am.J.Clin.Nutr., 21(7):746, 1968.
Ibid, 21:743, 1968.
Willis, G.C. and Fishman, S. Can.Med.Assn.J., 72:500, 1955.
Uhl, E. Am.J.Clin.Nutr., 6:146, 1958.
Begum, A. and Pererira, S. Brit.J.Nutr., 23(4):905, 1969.
Perera, W.D.A. and Reddy, V. Indian J.Med.Res., 59(6):961, 1971.
Fry, P.C. Nutr.Rep.Int., 6:99, 1972.
Manalo, R. and Jones, J.L. Am.J.Clin.Nutr., 18:339, 1966.
Oomen, H.A.P.C. Trop.Geogr.Med., 19(1):31, 1967.
Seelig, M.S. Am.J.Clin.Nutr. 14:342, 1964.
Organic Food Mktg. 5(8):2, 1974.
Drasar, B.S. and Hill, M.J. Am.J.Clin.Nutr., 25:1394, 1973.
Bishop, J.E. Wall Street Journal, October 23, 1973.
Kittler, G.D. "Control for Cancer," Warner, 1963.
Samson, E.I. Vrach, Delo, 12:33, 1971.
Isyeyev, M.K. Pediat.Akush.Hinekol., 32(2):41, 1970.
Gries, Christian L., J.Nutr., 102:1259, 1972.
Carre, L., et al. Nutr.Dieta. 11(4):241, 1969.
Guthrie, H.A. Op.Cit., p. 260.
Harris, P.L. and Embree, N.D. Am.J.Clin.Nutr., 13:385, 1963.
White, H.G. J.Am.Diet, Assoc., 55:33, 1969.